The Proof
Successes with cellular nutrients confirm
vitamin research findings

D090300?

The Proof

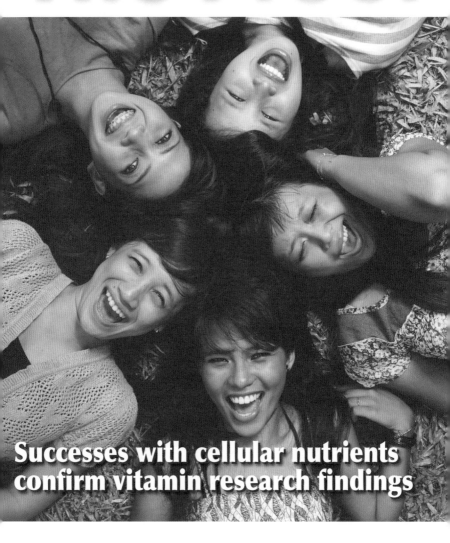

Successes with cellular nutrients confirm vitamin research findings

Dr. Rath Health Foundation

The Proof –
Successes with cellular nutrients confirm vitamin research findings

1st edition

© 2011 Dr. Matthias Rath

Distribution:
Dr. Rath Education Services B.V.
Postbus 656
NL-6400 AR Heerlen

Tel.:   0031-457-111 222
Fax: 0031-457-111 229

email   info@rath-eduserv.com
          books@rath-eduserv.com
website: www.rath-eduserv.com

All rights reserved. Published by the Dr. Rath Health Foundation. Single pages of this book can be copied for private and non-commercial purposes. Any direct or indirect commercial use of this book or parts thereof in any form is strictly prohibited without written permission from the authors.

For legal reasons we are obliged to issue the following statement:

This book does not aim to replace medical consultation with a doctor. In relation to health concerns the reader should consult a doctor or therapist, especially where symptoms of illness require medical diagnosis or treatment. The authors, the publisher and the publishing company cannot accept liability should side effects arise in direct or indirect consequence of the recommendations in this book.

The Proof

Successes with cellular nutrients confirm vitamin research findings

CONTENT

Foreword

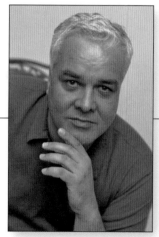

Dr. Matthias Rath

Cancer is no longer a death sentence!

The scientific foundations for ending the cancer epidemic have been described in detail in the book "Victory Over Cancer", which has already been translated into numerous languages.

The present book, "The Proof", now documents accounts by patients who have put their faith in these scientifically founded natural medical approaches. Most of these patients have been living a normal life for many years now – without suffering the agonies of chemotherapy, radiotherapy or other desperate measures used in orthodox cancer treatment.

The reports by cancer patients which we have compiled here document better than any clinical study the historic breakthrough that we are currently witnessing in this field of medicine – the transformation that is creating a world without fear of the "cancer" diagnosis.

The letters published here are representative of many hundreds of others received from cancer patients who wish to pass on to others – to you - their experiences with this disease.

The patients describe their "journey", from the terror of the first moment when they receive the cancer diagnosis, followed by pressure put on them by doctors to subject themselves at all costs to chemo- and radiotherapy, then their battles with themselves about the right course of action through to finding the courage to say "No" to systematic poisoning of their body – and finally the realization that they had made the right choice!

Naturally this book does not hold out the promise to readers that micronutrients – or cellular nutrients as we call them – can heal all types of cancer. In particular this will not be possible if the cancer is already far advanced or if numerous cycles of chemotherapy have severely damaged or even destroyed a patient's own immune system.

I know of no other research institute in recent years that has published more scientific studies on breakthroughs in natural cancer treatment than our research institute in California. These studies have been published online and are freely available at **www.cancer-free-world.org/scientific_facts/index.php** .

The momentum built up by the intensity of this fundamental scientific research has ensured that a large number of major clinical studies on cellular nutrients in relation to cancer are now being carried out at leading research centres and university clinics.

As you read this book, over a hundred such clinical studies are underway in the USA alone. It is foreseeable that within a few years cancer will change from being a "death sentence" to a treatable – and above all avoidable – disease.

The only interest group that still opposes the breathtaking prospect of a "world without cancer" is the pharma lobby with its billion-dollar investment in the "chemo" business. We must therefore recognize that the right to live in a world free of cancer is not going to be handed to us on a plate. We are going to have to work hard to achieve it.

If you wish to play a part in this great task, you will need to get all the information you can. If you do not already know it, you should read the book, "Victory Over Cancer". Part 1 of this book sets out the basic scientific information in an accessible way, and part 2 explains why you have not yet heard about this breakthrough.

It is self-evident that we cannot achieve this important goal of a "world without cancer" as isolated individuals. This is why we have launched an initiative in which all who wish to achieve this goal with us can work together. You will find further information on this at the website listed below. If you can see your way to doing this, you could found an initiative in your locality, to make your town or city a "cancer-free" zone.

I invite you to join us in this common endeavor. We should do this for ourselves, our children, and for all future generations.

The time to act is now!

Cordially yours,
Dr. Matthias Rath

www.cancer-free-world.org

Important notes

Some of the letters published here, from patients to Dr. Rath, were abbreviated for reasons of space. Every single letter, in the form published here, received its author's renewed confirmation and approval in the form of a signature.

Each patient also signed a declaration of agreement to publish. As the publishers of this book we guarantee the authenticity of all reports and letters reprinted here, specifically also in cases where – to protect privacy – we were asked to remove the patient's full name.

Many users of cellular nutrients also submitted their full medical records to us. We have printed copies here of some of these medical reports and x-rays in order to ensure that readers can understand this important documentation without medical knowledge.

If these reports give you pause for thought, and if you think that they might help people in your family circle, or your friends and acquaintances, or also your neighbors and people in your local community or area, then do pass this documentation on.

**By doing so you will be helping others,
and possibly even saving lives!**

What is cancer?

All cells, even healthy ones, that wish to migrate through the body, have to first dissolve the surrounding connective tissue consisting of a dense network of collagen fibres (connective tissue matrix). For this purpose cells can secrete special enzymes capable of digesting this collagen matrix.

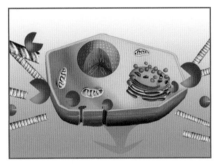

Cancer cells produce unlimited amounts of enzymes that enable them to spread and migrate. Further information on this can be found in the book, "Victory Over Cancer".

Under normal conditions, certain cells already use the same mechanism – the ovum, for instance, at ovulation, or the white blood corpuscles when 'migrating' to the site of an infection. When whole organs, too, are reconfigured - for example the womb during pregnancy or the female breast while breast-feeding – this occurs through controlled tissue breakdown and subsequent resynthesis. Under normal (physiological) conditions, the production and activity of these enzymes is carefully controlled so that they are only active for a short period, thus preventing continuous breakdown of collagen and permanent damage to tissue.

Unlike these normal, physiological processes, the control function is lost in the case of cancer cells. Not only do they multiply without hindrance but they also continually produce these enzymes that attack and destroy surrounding connective tissue. The degree of aggression of a malignant tumor is dependant primarily on the quantity of collagen-digesting enzymes produced.

All cancer cells – irrespective of their origin – produce large quantities of these enzymes, leading to destruction of surrounding connective tissue. With the aid of these "cutting tools", the cancer cells release themselves from the tumor and migrate into other organs via the blood or lymph systems – a process known as metastasis.

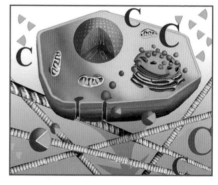

Two important dietary supplements are vitamin C and lysine, neither of which can be produced by the body itself. Lysine (green wedges) blocks the collagen-digesting enzymes, thus hindering decomposition. Vitamin C, by contrast, promotes the development of connective tissue.

Orthodox cancer treatment and its side effects

Cancer has been treated for decades by standard methods such as surgery, chemotherapy and radiotherapy. The most commonly used forms of treatment – chemotherapy and radiotherapy – indiscriminately attack not only cancer cells but also healthy cells, which is why they are associated with severe side effects. The most common side effect is the growth of new cancer, since both chemo- and radiotherapy cause damage to genetic material (DNA).

Cellular nutrients can control decisive stages of cancer cell migration

Cellular nutrients can help inhibit the spread of cancer cells in four major ways:

1. They can inhibit the reproduction of cancer cells.

2. They can inhibit the spread of cancer cells, a precondition of metastasis.

3. They can inhibit the formation of tumor blood vessels by means of which the growing tumor is nourished

4. They can kill cancer cells.

Important cellular nutrients for combating cancer
Important substances and their functions:

Vitamin C
is needed for forming collagen and thus for connective tissue stability. Studies at the US National Institutes of Health (NIH) have shown that vitamin C at high concentrations can kill cancer cells **without** impairing healthy cells.

Lysine and Proline
are natural amino acids which primarily serve as constituents of collagen molecules and thus support tissue stability. They are also capable of at least partially inhibiting the collagen-digesting enzymes and thus counteracting the unhindered spread of cancer cells.

Polyphenols
are likewise capable of inhibiting the activity of collagen-digesting enzymes, and thus combat the spread of cancer cells.

N-acetyl cysteine (NAC)
is a strong anti-oxidant and important for the synthesis of glutathione, another effective anti-oxidant.

Arginine
improves the action of the immune system and inhibits the reproduction of cancer cells.

Selenium
is an important component of the anti-oxidative defense system and protects cells against toxins. It can also inhibit the growth of tumor cells.

Specific plant extracts
have important protective functions for the human body, especially as a natural means to counteract cell mutation and cancer, due to their strong anti-oxidative properties and their ability to combat bacteria, viruses and other harmful agents.

Common types of cancer

In their book, "Victory Over Cancer", Dr. Matthias Rath and Dr. Aleksandra Niedzwiecki explain why cancer is especially common in organs in which breakdown of connective tissue already occurs under normal physiological conditions.

The reproductive organs are the first such organ group, susceptible to cancer types that include breast cancer, ovarian cancer, uterine cancer, cervical cancer, testicular cancer and prostate cancer.

Below you will first find a few examples of people affected by these types of cancer, who report here on their experiences with cellular nutrients.

Breast cancer

Ovarian cancer

Uterine cancer

Cervical cancer

Testicular cancer

Prostate cancer

Leukemia

Breast cancer

Dear Dr. Rath

I thank my lucky stars every day that I found out about Cellular Medicine.

In 2002, at the age of 60, I stopped working due to heart arrhythmia and high blood pressure.

These complaints arose from long periods of stress. For two long years I took pharma pills but my condition did not improve.

By now my pulse rate had fallen to 35 bpm, and 49 after exertion. Then I remembered the lecture of yours I had attended years before in Hamburg, and I started to take cellular nutrients.

After a week I already felt a slight improvement in the heart arrhythmia. After a month it had almost disappeared. Then I went to my GP and she found that my blood pressure and pulse rate had also improved. She was astonished and said, "This has nothing to do with the pills you're taking." At this I told her about Cellular Medicine and she was pleasantly surprised.

In 2008, during a routine mammogram, a small cancerous tumor was found. My family urged me to have an operation: a small piece was removed from my breast and a few lymph nodes in my armpit.

Following this I was meant to take pharma pills for five years to prevent a recurrence of cancer, and also to receive precautionary radiotherapy – but I categorically refused.

I am very pleased that I did so, for today I am in the best of health. No cancer ever recurred, for I kept using cellular nutrients throughout.

I have absolute confidence in cellular nutrients, and my health could not be better!

Warm and healthy greetings
Ilse Goersch

Breast cancer

Dear Dr. Rath

My name is Bozena Herzner. During an examination on 28.3.2005, a mammary carcinoma was found in my breast, and this was confirmed in mammograms and blood tests on 6.4.2005 and 12.4.2005. No metastases were found.

After diagnosis I underwent breast-conserving surgery. According to my medical records, on removal the carcinoma was found to be deeply embedded within healthy tissue. I dispensed with all chemo- and radiotherapy, and also with hormone-inhibiting medicines. Directly after surgery I took cellular nutrients and am still taking them to this day.

Further mammograms on 23.3.2006 and 15.11.2006 showed that no secondary carcinoma developed, nor did any relapse occur.

Besides using cellular nutrients I also changed my diet. I started with food combining and I eat only organic food. I attribute my health to all these measures.

My follow-up care chart from 2005 to 2011 shows that no subsequent deterioration occurred in my state of health.

I am glad that I pursued my own path, and I'd like to encourage others to do the same!

Yours sincerely

Bozena Herzner

Medical reports for Mrs Herzner are documented on the following pages.

Medical report for Bozena Herzner dated 6.4.2005, confirming that she had breast cancer.

28/04 2005 10:43 FAX

FROM: Gemeinschaftspraxis Pathologen   TO: PAGE: 1 OF 1

GEMEINSCHAFTS-PRAXIS PATHOLOGIE

Eingang: 6.04.2005 la
Patient:
Herzner
Bozena

Untersuchung

Ausgang: 6.04.2005

Art/Herkunft des Materials - **Erneuter Ausdruck am 11.04.05 mit Nachtrag**
Mammastanzbiopsie rechts

Histopathologische Begutachtung:

Drei Stanzanteile zusammen 2,0 cm mit Mammaparenchym und in allen drei
Stanzen ausgedehnten Infiltraten eines teils tubulär, teils solide wachsen-
den Tumorgewebes in einem desmoplastischen Stroma. Die Tumorzellen mäßig
polymorph mit einzelnen atypischen Mitosefiguren. Fokal fragliche intraduk-
tale Anteile mit Nekrose. Tumorzellen z. T. in Spalten.

BEURTEILUNG:
Mammastanze rechts mit einem invasiv-duktalen **Mammakarzinom** (G2, Score 6)
mit Verdacht auf Lymphangiosis carcinomatosa.

Befundkategorie nach den Richtlinien des NHS Brustscreening-Programms
(Großbritannien): B5

Das Ergebnis der immunhistochemischen Untersuchung folgt als Nachtrag.

NACHTRAG (Ausgang am 11.04.05):

Immunhistochemischer Hormonrezeptorstatus:
positiv (Östrogen mit einem immunreaktiven Score (IRS) von 9 bei 70 % posi-
tiven Zellen und Progesteron mit einem IRS von 9 bei 60 % postiven Zellen
(IRS-Bereich: 0 bis 12)).
HER2neu-Überexpression (Dako): negativ Score 0 (bei regulärer Reaktion im
mitgeführten Multiblock-Kontrollpräparat).

(Bericht per EDV als Telefax aufbereitet und daher nicht unterschrieben)

Medical report for Bozena Herzner, dated 6.4.2005 and lab report dated 20.4.2005. Diagnosis: Breast cancer.

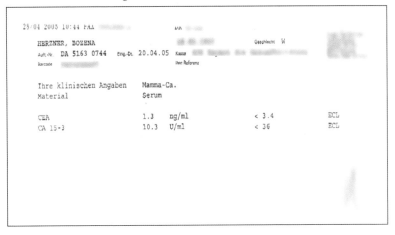

28/04 2005 10:44 FAX		DR			
HERZNER, BOZENA			Geschlecht W		
Auft.-Nr. DA 5163 0744	Eing.-Dt. 20.04.05	Kasse			
Barcode		Ihre Referenz			
Ihre klinischen Angaben	Mamma-Ca.				
Material	Serum				
CEA	1.3	ng/ml	< 3.4	ECL	
CA 15-3	10.3	U/ml	< 36	ECL	

CEA and CA are so-called "tumor markers" measured in the blood.

Assessment: Mammary screening of right side showed invasive ductal mammary carcinoma (G2, score 6).

Medical report for Bozena Herzner, dated 15.3.2006, confirming that no breast cancer can be detected.

Zentrum für Microdosis-Mammographie
Privatpraxis

Zentrum für Microdosis-Mammographie •

nachrichtlich an Pat.

München, den 23.03.06

Digitale Microdosis-Mammographie bds. in zwei Ebenen am 15.3.06

Sehr geehrter Herr Kollege

ich berichte Ihnen heute über Ihre Patientin Frau **Bozena Herzner,**

Indikation und Anamnese: Zustand nach Mamma-Ca. rechts und OP 2005. Kontrollmammographie, Tumorausschluss.

Palpation und Inspektion: inspektorisch und palpatorisch keine Auffälligkeiten. Narbe rechts reizlos. Kleinknotige Einlagerungen bds..

Microdosis Mammographie bds.: es findet sich sehr dichtes Drüsengewebe. Es zeigen sich insgesamt inhomogene Strukturen. Im Bereich der Narbe rechts keine Auffälligkeiten. Eine Verdichtungsstruktur links auf der CC-Aufnahme zentral ist auf den Voraufnahmen von 2005 in gleicher Weise erkennbar. Ansonsten keine weiteren Auffälligkeiten.

Beurteilung: bei Zustand nach Mamma-Ca. rechts und OP jetzt kein Hinweis auf ein Zweitkarzinom oder Rezidiv.

links: BIRADS II, gesamt: ACR IV.

Procedere: es wird eine Kontrollmammographie und –sonographie in etwa 6 Monat   hlen. Die Patientin ist über das weitere Procedere informiert.

Mit freundlichen kollegialen Grüßen

Ihre Dr. med.

Assessment: Following mammary carcinoma on right side and surgery, no further indication of secondary carcinoma or relapse.

Medical report for Bozena Herzner, dated 14.11.2006,
likewise confirming that no breast cancer can be detected.

ZENTRUM FÜR
MICRODOSIS-MAMMOGRAPHIE

- Privatpraxis -

Dr. med.
Zentrum für Microdosis-Mammographie   )r. med.
Dr. med.
Frau   Dr. med.

, 15.11.2006
415228/Zo/rtg.

Digitale Microdosis-Mammographie beidseits in zwei Ebenen
und hochauflösende Mammasonographie bds. sowie Sonographie beider Axillen im
Powerdopplermodus am 14.11.2006

Sehr geehrte Frau

ich berichte Ihnen heute über Ihre Untersuchung.

Indikation und Anamnese: Mamma-Ca. rechts. Zustand nach Tumorexstirpation eines
Mamma-Ca. gegen 11 Uhr brustwandnah 04/05 ohne Radiatio oder Chemotherapie.

Klinischer Untersuchungsbefund: Bei der Inspektion reizlose Narbe rechts oben außen
gegen 11 Uhr, palpatorisch unauffällig rechtsseitig, linksseitig tastet man gegen 1 Uhr einen
mobilen, ganz oberflächlich gelegenen Knoten von knapp 1 cm Größe.

Microdosis Mammographie bds.: Mammographisch stellt sich eine dichte Mamma dar mit
unauffälligem Drüsengewebe. Cutisverdickung und zarte narbige Einlagerungen rechts
oben außen. Auf der Oblique-Aufnahme links vor der vorderen Axillarlinie stellt sich ein
ovaler, glatt begrenzter Knoten von knapp 1 cm Größe dar. Nirgends umschriebener
Mikrokalk. Die auf der Voraufnahme beschriebene Verdichtung im CC-Strahlengang löst
sich heute auf.

Sonographie bds. sowie Axillen bds. im Powerdopplermodus: Sonographisch im
Narbengebiet kein Hinweis für ein Rezidiv. Beidseits echoreiche Strukturen im Sinne von
Drüsengewebe; links gegen 1 Uhr ein ovaler, horizontal wachsender areflektiver, glatt
begrenzter Herd. Kollateralphänomen, dorsale Schallverstärkung. Bei Powerdoppler-
sonographie keine Durchblutung, also im Sinne einer Zyste. Axillae frei.

Beurteilung: Zustand nach Tumorexstirpation rechts, zarte narbige Einlagerung gegen 11
Uhr. Links gegen 1 Uhr blande Zyste. Kein Malignomverdacht.

No suspected malignant tumor.

25

Breast cancer

Dear Dr. Rath

I am very pleased to write to you to report on my experiences with cellular nutrients.

I heard about Cellular Medicine by chance in 2004. Since I felt very weakened by breast surgery, and chemo- and radiotherapy in 2000, as well as by a borreliosis infection in 2003, which may not have been properly treated, I saw Cellular Medicine as an opportunity to improve my health by natural means.

In February 2004 I attended an information event on Cellular Medicine in Leipzig, and learned many interesting things about this approach. I was struck by the clear presentations and accessible information material, with reports from grateful patients who had regained their health, and so I immediately started taking cellular nutrients. Complemented by regular saunas, swimming, Nordic walking and fitness training, my current good state of health remains stable.

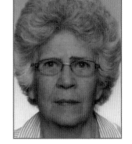

Despite my 77 years I am now very happy, and pleased at the success achieved by the Health Alliance. I very much hope you will gain greater publicity, and an ultimate victory over the rigid, conventional pharmaceutical industry. I feel renewed gratitude every day that I heard about your work.

Yours sincerely

Helga-Maria Leipnitz

Medical report for Helga-Maria Leipnitz, dated 10.8.2011, confirming the absence of any breast cancer.

Helga-Maria Leipnitz, geb.am ▓▓ ▓▓ *Nachdruck*

Befund vom 10.08.2011, Befund freigegeben   Diktierer: ▓▓ **Freigeber:** ▓▓
zu Maßnahmen
MXUSBS vom 03.08.2011 12:57
MXBS vom 03.08.2011 11:39

Überweiser: ▓▓ ▓▓ **Dr. med.**

Mammographie bds. und Mamma-Sonographie bds. vom 03.08.2011:

Klinik:
Z.n. BET li. 12/99 mit Axilladissektion und Radiochemotherapie. Einnahme von Tamoxifen bzw. Femara bis 2007. Z.n. PE re. 12/99 und VB li. 2004, beides mit benignem Ergebnis. Familienanamnese leer.
Aktuell keine Hormonsubstitution. Die Pat. berichtet über diffuse Schmerzen in der li. Brust, die schon immer gelegentlich, jetzt wohl durch vermehrten Sport etwas verstärkt sind. Zusätzlich berichtet sie über eine chron. Borreliose.

Inspektion und Palpation:
Die Narben li. oben außen sowie in der li. Axillae bei Z.n. BET sowie die Narbe re. oben außen bei Z.n. PE stellen sich reizlos dar. Das Narbenareal li. oben außen tastet sich dezent dichter als das übrige Brustgewebe – laut Pat. so seit BET und im Wesentlichen unverändert. Bds. lassen sich darüber hinaus keine umschriebenen, suspekten Tastbefunde erheben. Keine patholog. LK-Schwellung. Keine Sekretion. Kein Ekzem. Keine Einziehungen.

Mammographie:
Es liegen VA vom 29.06.10 vor.
Es zeigt sich im Wesentlichen unverändert eine partielle Involution mit kleinfleckig konfiguriertem Restdrüsengewebe. Re. zeigt sich präpektoral, leicht oben auf der Quadrantengrenze, eine flaue, drüsengewebsisodense Verdichtung, die sich bereits in VA von 2001 abgrenzen lässt und dazu im Wesentlichen unverändert erscheint – a.e. handelt es sich um eine Drüsengewebsinsel. Li. zeigen sich zentral im hinteren Brustdrittel grobe Verkalkungen – a.e. handelt es sich um ein regressiv verkalkendes Fibroadenom. Bds. zeigen sich einzelne, kleine unauffällig erscheinende Mikroverkalkungen. Unauffällige LK axillär re. Bds. kein Nachweis malignomsuspekter Mikroverkalkungen. Diskrete, residuelle Cutisverdickung li. bei Z.n. BET.

Mammasonographie:
In der ergänzenden Mammasonographie zeigt sich li. oben, leicht innen eine quer ovale, scharf begrenzte, echoarme Struktur, randständig mit deutlicher Schallauslöschung – im Vergleich zur VU im Wesentlichen unverändert erscheinend und a.e. einem z.T. verkalkten Fibroadenom entsprechend. Re. unten außen findet sich eine kleine quer ovale, scharf begrenzte echoarme Struktur von etwa 2 x 4 x 5 mm Größe – a.e. handelt es sich um eine kleine Zyste. Bds. kein Nachweis umschriebener malignomsuspekter Läsionen. Die Axillae stellen sich beide unauffällig dar.

Beurteilung:
Derzeit kein Anhalt für Malignität.
Bei fehlenden klin. Auffälligkeiten wird eine Kontrolle in ca. 1 Jahr empfohlen.
Klassifikation: ACR III, BIRADS 2.

Mit freundlichen Grüßen

OA Dr. med. ▓▓   ▓▓   ▓▓
FA f. Diagn. Radiologie   Arzt   Arzt

Assessment: Currently no reason to suspect malignancy.

Breast cancer

Dear Dr. Rath

I fell ill with breast cancer in May 2007: the tumor was already 1.8 centimetres in size. Fortunately I knew someone who had herself had breast cancer, and had found cellular nutrients to be an excellent remedy. From her I obtained information material including a DVD with your series of lectures from 2007. The understandable, logical explanations helped me decide to undergo surgery to remove the tumor and then start immediately with a course of cellular nutrient treatment.

The tumor was removed at Berlin's Charité Hospital. Naturally I was advised to have radio- and chemotherapy. I refused both and instead turned to cellular nutrients. None of the doctors agreed with this plan, of course, but they accepted my decision.

A few days after the operation I received the diagnosis that the tumor was a so-called inflammatory carcinoma – an inflammatory form of cancer with a very poor prognosis due to its metastasising mechanism. However, I kept to my decision. My gynaecologist was opposed to this.

Four years later, on 31 May 2011, I went for a check-up. My doctor said that he could find 'nothing of concern'. My good state of health, due to cellular nutrients, left me optimistic throughout that I had made the right decision. And confirmation of this by the medical examination made this day the happiest of my life.

It is high time that I thanked you and your whole team, Dr. Rath, for your great endeavours and for the incalculable value of insights that have saved me much suffering and literally saved my life.

Yours sincerely
G.M.

Dear Dr. Rath

Ten years ago I was diagnosed with breast cancer that had also gone into the lymph nodes. Not for a moment did I contemplate amputation of the breast or chemotherapy.

I decided instead to take natural cellular nutrients, which I have been using successfully to this day. I also received mistletoe injections and took anti-oestrogens for three years, and homeopathic remedies. So far there has been no recurrence of cancer.

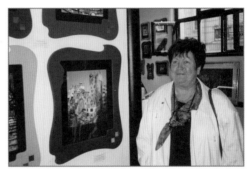

I feel well – except for the fact that I was given a new knee in May 2011, and had to take painkillers and anti-inflammatory medicines for five weeks. I believe that cellular nutrients helped me recover from the knee operation and get fit again quickly.

Yours sincerely
Erika Raetzer

Breast cancer

My name is Bärbel Saliger. Twelve years ago, in January, I thought my life was at an end. The diagnosis of breast cancer pulled the rug out from under my feet.

Heavy chemotherapy sessions made me a wheelchair invalid. Then there were financial problems as well, and I was battling alone since the husband who had sworn to love me could no longer cope with me in the low state chemotherapy left me in. With just one breast he no longer considered me a woman. I could have had breast reconstruction, but I always say: If some-one loves me, they will accept me as I am.

Now someone may ask: heavy chemo, wheelchair – how come she's thriving now and looks so well?

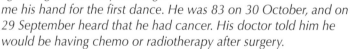

Since 2001 I have been taking cellu-lar nutrients. After only three weeks, the pains in my legs faded. After a month I said: "Cheerio wheelchair!"

In March 2002 I celebrated my birthday with my whole family. After agonising months, my father gave me his hand for the first dance. He was 83 on 30 October, and on 29 September heard that he had cancer. His doctor told him he would be having chemo or radiotherapy after surgery.

My father immediately refused this, relating the bad experiences I had gone through with these forms of treatment. He had watched me suffering. He decided to take cellular nutrients, for he too had repeatedly been astonished at the way I was getting my life back after such difficult times.

For my 60th birthday we will both open the dance. And there will be another special reason for celebration: in February my daughter gave me the gift of my first grandchild.

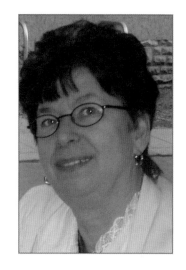

I can only say, to anyone who is still doubtful about Dr. Rath and his team, that chemical concoctions are only good for those who make money from them. I thank you, Dr. Rath and your team.

I also want to thank Werner Pilniok and his wife who encouraged me to take the right course of action at the time, and who remain my very good friends.

With warmest regards, your Bärbel Saliger

Breast cancer

Dear ladies and gentlemen

In May 2007 I received the greatest shock of my 66 years. I had felt a lump in my breast for a while. My naturopath sent me to the gynaecologist, who in turn sent me to the hospital. All the preliminary tests, and a biopsy, showed that the lump in my right breast was a cancerous tumor, measuring around 3 centimetres – it was slow-growing and not aggressive.

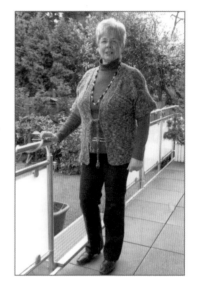

The subsequent breast-conserving operation with removal of the tumor and surrounding tissue went well, without complications. Before surgery, and after it too, my general state of health was very good. All tests and my bloodcount were in order. After my 8-day stay in the hospital, I was told that follow-up care would include three cycles of chemotherapy and 28 radiotherapy sessions.

As soon as I knew that I had breast cancer I was absolutely clear that I would not submit to chemotherapy or radiation treatment. My decision met with fierce opposition from the doctors at the hospital. My husband was present at all consultations and supported my decision. When we asked about other forms of follow-up care, the doctors were unable to offer anything else!

I was therefore discharged from hospital and was initially happy and relieved that I had got rid of the tumor. I was clear that my 'follow-up care' would be based on Cellular Medicine; and I have been taking cellular nutrients regularly ever since.

To sum up: All regular check-ups since then have shown positive results, with no sign of cancer. Even a major follow-up examination in the hospital in February 2011, including ultrasound and a rigorous blood test, was absolutely fine – to the doctors' astonishment – with no pathological findings.

The doctors were so surprised that they had the tests repeated twice by various different specialists in the breast cancer department.

I have frequently passed onto others my experiences with Cellular Medicine. These patients too reported back to me on their outstanding success and confirmed their recovery.

Since I and my family are thriving on our daily intake of cellular nutrients, and feel well, we can recommend this mode of precautionary healthcare with a very good conscience.

In the hope that we will continue to maintain our good health for many years to come, I remain

yours, with best regards
Rita Strauch

Frau Strauch's medical report is documented on the following page

Medical reported for Rita Strauch, dated 30.5.2007, confirming breast cancer diagnosis.

**Frauenklinik und
Zentrum für Reproduktionsmedizin**

Herr

**Evangelisches
Krankenhaus**

Sehr geehrter Herr Kollege,

**Akademisches
Lehrkrankenhaus
der Universität**

wir berichten Ihnen über Ihre Patientin,
Frau Rita <u>Strauch</u>, geb. am
wohnhaft
die sich vom 23.05.2007 bis zum 31.05.2007 in unserer stationären
Behandlung befand.

Telefon
Durchwahl
Telefax
www.   .de

31.05..2007 /

<u>**Diagnose:**</u>	Mammakarzinom rechts
<u>**Tumorstadium:**</u>	pT2, G2, pN1 (1/16), L1, V0, R
<u>**Rezeptorstatus:**</u>	ER:12, PR:12, Her2neu: +
<u>**Histologie:**</u>	wurde Ihnen bereits zugefaxt / s.o.
<u>**Therapie:**</u>	Operativ:16.05.2007: Stanze rechts 24.05.2007: Mamma-TE + Axilladissektion rechts
<u>**Verlauf:**</u>	Der intra- und postoperative Verlauf gestaltete sich komplikationslos.
<u>**Staging:**</u>	**Thorax: o.B.** **Lebersonographie: o.B.** **Knochenscan**: degenrative Veränderungen, keine metastasenverdächtigen Herde

Ergebnis der Tumorkonferenz vom: 30.05.2007: Bei o.g. Tumorformel wird der Patientin eine
systemische Therapie mit 3 Zyklen FEC/ 3 Zyklen Taxotere empfohlen Bei Z.n. BET sollte die
Radiatio der Brust erfolgen. Der Rezeptorstatus steht bei auswärts durchgeführter Stanzbiopsie
noch aus. Ggfls ist eine antihormonelle Therapie indiziert.

Nach intensiver Aufklärung und Beratung auch mit den niedergelassenen Kollegen lehnt die
Patientin eine Chemotherapie ab. Eine Vorstellung zur Planung der Radiatio wurde mit ihr für
den 14.06. vereinbart.
Mit freundlichem Gruß!

Prof. Dr. med.   Dr.
Chefarzt   Ltd. Oberarzt   Stationsarzt

Diagnosis: Right-side mammary carcinoma

Stand 12/2004

DOKUMENTIERTE PATIENTENAUFKLÄRUNG

Basisinformation zum ärztlichen Aufklärungsgespräch

Klinikeindruck/Stempel

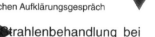

Strahlenbehandlung bei Brustkrebs

- ☒ nach brusterhaltender Operation
- ☐ nach Brustentfernung (Mastektomie)
- ☐ Rückfallbehandlung (Rezidiv)
- ☒ Bestrahlung nur Brustdrüse
- ☐ Bestrahlung Brustdrüse und Lymphabflussstationen
  - ☐ axillär
  - ☐ parasternal
  - ☐ supraclaviculär
- ☒ Bestrahlung
  - ☐ links
  - ☒ rechts
  - ☐ beidseitig

Patientendaten/Aufkleber

Fr. Strauch, Rita * 09.06.1941

Liebe Patientin, lieber Patient,

zu Ihrer Behandlung gibt es mehrere Möglichkeiten, nämlich Operation, Strahlentherapie, Hormontherapie und zytostatische Chemotherapie, die auch miteinander kombiniert werden können. Nach gewissenhafter Prüfung empfehlen wir jetzt die Strahlentherapie. Sie bietet Ihnen die besten Heilungschancen.
Vor der Behandlung wird die Ärztin/der Arzt (im Folgenden nur Arzt) mit Ihnen über Notwendigkeit und Durchführung der geplanten Maßnahme sprechen. Sie müssen typische Risiken und Folgen kennen, damit Sie sich eine Meinung bilden und in die Behandlung einwilligen können. Dieses Aufklärungsblatt soll das Gespräch unterstützen und helfen, die für Sie wichtigsten Belange zu besprechen und zu dokumentieren.

Was sollten Sie über eine Strahlenbehandlung wissen?

Zur Strahlenbehandlung verwenden wir sogenannte **ionisierende Strahlen**. Diese sind im Gegensatz zu anderen Strahlungsarten, z.B. Sonnen-, Wärmeoder Laserstrahlen, in der Lage, die kleinsten Bausteine unseres Körpers (Atome und Moleküle) in ihrer Struktur zu verändern (Ionisation); dies führt zu Folgen in den kranken und gesunden Körpergeweben. Der Erfolg der Behandlung hängt davon ab, wie gut das kranke Gewebe reagiert und das gesunde Gewebe die Strahlen verträgt.

Strahlen wirken nur in dem zu behandelnden Bereich. In Frage kommen grundsätzlich Röntgen-, Gamma- oder Teilchenstrahlen (z.B. Elektronen). Diese sollen krankhaft veränderte Zellen gezielt zerstören. Gelingt dies, bildet sich die Geschwulst entweder völlig zurück, verkleinert sich deutlich oder stellt zumindest ihr Wachstum ein.

Welche Vorbereitungen sind nötig?

Zunächst beurteilt der Arzt die Ausbreitung Ihrer Tumorerkrankung durch körperliche Untersuchung sowie mit speziellen bildgebenden Verfahren (z.B. Röntgen, Ultraschall, Computer- und Kernspin-Tomographie). Ggf. werden die Befunde von einer vorangegangenen Operation und die feingewebliche Beurteilung herangezogen, z.B. über die Beschaffenheit der Operationsgrenzen und der entfernten Lymphknoten. Dann legt der Arzt das zu bestrahlende Zielgebiet fest.

Häufig werden Hilfsmittel angefertigt, die die exakte Lage Ihres Körpers bei den täglichen Bestrahlungen sicherstellen. Diese sogenannten **Lagerungshilfen** gewährleisten, dass das Zielgebiet immer genau getroffen wird und sichern damit den Behandlungserfolg.

Die günstigsten Eintrittspforten für die Bestrahlungen findet der Arzt am Computer- und Kernspin-Tomographen, auch mit Hilfe eines speziellen Röntgengerätes (**Therapie-Simulator**). Werden zur Planung der Strahlenbehandlung **Röntgenkontrastmittel** in die Vene eingespritzt, können in seltenen Fällen Unverträglichkeitsreaktionen auftreten, z.B. an der Haut, den Atmungsorganen, den Nieren, am Nerven- und Herz-Kreislaufsystem. Schwere lebensbedrohliche Zwischenfälle sind aber sehr selten.

Für gewöhnlich wird das zu behandelnde Zielgebiet über verschiedene Strahlrichtungen angegangen, um das gesunde Gewebe bestmöglich schonen zu können. Dazu tragen auch Abdeckungen aus strahlenundurchlässigem Material bei, die eigens für

Frau Strauch also kindly sent her "patient information sheet" – a document that has to be signed by every patient before radiotherapy can be carried out. The side effects listed in it, including the development of further cancer (which it describes as "secondary growth" to make it seem less important), give a striking sense of the current impasse in which modern cancer treatment finds itself. (The full sheet is available).

Breast cancer

Dear Dr. Rath

The continual good health I have enjoyed in recent years has led me to update an earlier letter I sent you about my experiences, and send it to you once again.

I am now 64, and almost twelve years have passed since the "breast cancer" diagnosis, followed by surgery, chemo- and radio-therapy. I am still well – though that hardly does justice to it. In fact I am even better than I was nine, ten and more years ago!

When I received the "breast cancer" diagnosis in 1999 I felt despair, and my consultants' efforts to reassure me were of little help. Barely two years before this I had come through a complex gastric operation. Were things about to get even worse?

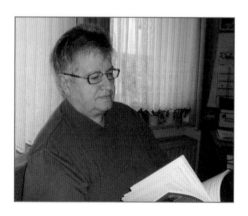

Fortunately all took a turn for the better – two books by you, Dr. Rath, made it easy for me to decide to start taking cellular nutrients alongside clinical treatment. I was able to avoid all the feared side effects of chemo- and radio-therapy by using cellu-lar nutrients. My hair didn't fall out but actually grew thicker – a fact that astonished my hairdresser.

This was in March 2000. In the years following my last chemother-apy treatment I stopped taking any pharmaceutical drugs, having decided I would rather be naturally well than pharma-sick!

In a few weeks' time it will be 2012. All medical examinations - tumor marker and blood tests in November 2011 – have been very satisfactory. Little aches and pains are fully under control, and I combat them by natural methods.

My husband and I have both long since recognized that there are natural alternatives to pharmaceutical drugs and conventional therapies. It really is high time that other people realized this, and took the opportunity to improve their lives. What I keep saying to people is this: Health isn't the be-all and end-all, but without it all's at an end!

And precisely for this reason we are going to keep working for a new, better health system, for the Health Alliance, and above all for you Dr. Rath!

Once again, Dr. Rath, we offer you our appreciation and thanks for your exemplary commitment and your battle to create a healthy world. As ever, we wish you and your research team continuing success with your socially responsible research work.

Warm greetings
Your Anna-Luise Korkowsky

Breast cancer

My name is Hannelore Wagner.

On 28 June 2007, as required by my health insurer, I went for a screening test (mammogram). Around 14 days later a radiologist sent me a message asking me to contact her.

At this second consultation the radiologist did an ultrasound scan and took a punch-biopsy tissue sample. She told me this would be examined by a pathologist and that I would receive the result in a few days. However, she said she already knew the lump was malignant.

This diagnosis was like a blow to the head. I just kept thinking: "I have cancer." The tears were streaming down my face as I drove home.

The following Tuesday I knew for certain: the lump in my breast was 7 millimetres in size. My gynaecologist advised me to have surgery as soon as possible. After thinking hard about it, I applied to a gynaecological clinic in Munich and underwent surgery there on 26 September 2007.

After a few days the doctor came to my bed and told me the pathologist had found no signs of cancer. She was unable to explain it. Once again I had to have a mammogram and magnetic resonance imaging. It turned out that the wrong lump had been removed! On the initial mammogram images there were two discernible lumps, and the malignant one was still there!

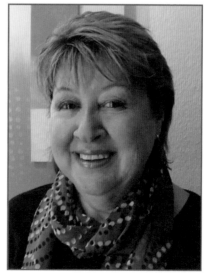

A few days later, after the second operation, I was discharged with notification that I would receive chemotherapy in the near future, and subsequently also radiotherapy. My gynaecologist explained what would happen. She said I would have to have five months of aggressive chemotherapy and then one month of radiotherapy.

However, I first wanted to try something else, since I had seen the effects of chemotherapy on my, sadly, late husband.

I had heard about cellular nutrients from my sister-in-law in 2003, and now immediately started to take them. From the first day onwards I have been feeling fine. That was four years ago, and I never regretted for a moment deciding against chemo- and radiotherapy.

I am proud and happy that instead I decided to take cellular nutrients, and would like to encourage everyone to do the same if they are diagnosed with cancer.

Medical reports and x-rays are attached.

**The medical report and
x-rays follow below.**

Medical report for Hannelore Wagner, dated 20.6.2007, confirming breast cancer.

FROM: Gemeinschaftspraxis Pathologen 08151/78420 TO: 0821555670 PAGE: 1 OF 1

PD Dr.
PD Dr.
Dr.
Dr.
Dr.

GEMEINSCHAFTS-PRAXIS PATHOLOGIE

- Tel 0   - Fax 0
Internet: www.   - Email: praxis@

Eingang: 20.08.2007 le
Patient:
Wagner
Hannelore

Dr. med.
Radiologin

Untersuchung HB07-49976

Ausgang: 20.08.2007   wg/lo

Art/Herkunft des Materials
Mammastanzbiopsie rechts

Histopathologische Begutachtung:

Vier zusammen 4 cm lange Zylinder eines Brustdrüsengewebes, das in allen vier Zylindern von einem epithelialen Tumor infltriert wird. Der Tumor wächst überwiegend in schmalen Trabekeln, in kleineren Abschnitten auch in tubulären Verbänden und setzt sich aus mittelgroßen Epithelien mit mäßig vergrößerten und polymorphen Kernen zusammen. Die Tubuli sind z.T. zirkulär um ortsständige Gangstrukturen angeordnet. Die mitotische Aktivität der Tumorzellen ist mittelgradig gesteigert (12-22 Mitosen pro 10 HPF bei 0,62 mm Gesichtsfelddurchmesser).

BEURTEILUNG:
Invasiv-ductales Mammakarzinom (G2/Score 6).

Befundkategorie nach den Richtlinien des NHS Brustscreening-Programms (Großbritannien): B5.

Immunhistologische Untersuchungen zur Frage ein   ptor-Positivität bzw. Her2neu-Überexpression sind eingeleitet worden,   eren Auswertung erfolgt ein Zweitbericht. Außerdem erfolgt eine e   Zweitbeurteilung im Rahmen des Mammographie-Screenings.

Dr.

(Eine interne Zweitbeurteilung erfolgte im Rahmen des Q   smanagements durch Dr.   )
Eine Kopie dieses Befundes geht an das Tumorzentrum

(Bericht per EDV als Telefax aufbereitet und daher nicht un   eben)

Assessment: Invasive ductal mammary carcinoma

X-ray for Hannelore Wagner, dated 28.6.2007, confirming breast cancer.

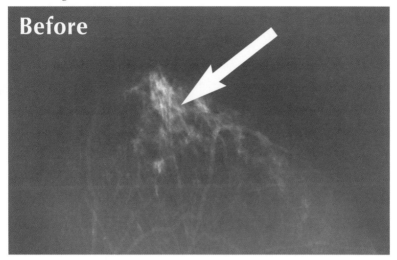

4 years later: X-ray for Hannelore Wagner, dated 24. 1. 2011, confirming that no breast cancer can be detected.

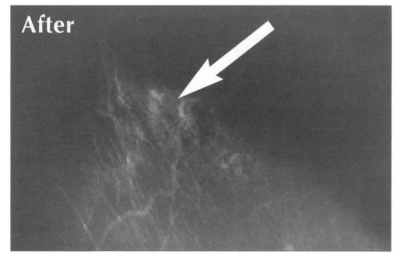

Breast cancer

Dear Dr. Rath

I am 64. In 2000 I felt a lump in my right breast, and breast cancer was subsequently diagnosed. In July 2000 the right breast was therefore removed completely, and chemotherapy began about two months later – a hellish experience, during which I felt I was wasting away.

Up to December 2000 I submitted to four cycles of chemotherapy and, in the following months, a total of 25 radiotherapy sessions. My immune system was radically weakened, and for a few days I could neither eat nor drink, so that by the end of February I needed to recover at a health spa.

Good friends then told me about cellular nutrients, and I started carefully studying books and brochures about it. All I read struck me as incredible – that entirely natural medical help was indeed available.

Since March 2001 I have been taking cellular nutrients every day. After just four weeks I found that I was recovering quickly from chemotherapy, and my immune system has stabilized, For me it was like a miracle to take something, at last, that was effective but had NO SIDE EFFECTS. It is not just that I am feeling very well, but the lab findings also give me a clean bill of health. I have conquered the cancer – and eleven years after the devastating diagnosis there are no longer any signs of it.

Since I started taking cellular nutrients, I have no longer caught flu or similar illnesses either, and still feel well. What more can one ask?

I also changed my diet and play sport regularly.

It is simply astonishing what a tough fight you have on your hands, Dr. Rath. I admire you and am very grateful.

With the very best wishes and regards
Your Marlies Schwietzer

Ovarian cancer

Dear ladies and gentlemen

In 2004, while searching on the internet, we became aware of Dr. Rath's findings in relation to various cellular nutrient compounds. My mother had been diagnosed with ovarian cancer in 2003. The specific diagnosis was: Fallopian tube cancer right side FIGO III c, ED 11/03.

After surgery at the end of 2003, my mother was to undergo chemotherapy in the context of a research study. Because of her poor health after the operation, and leg paralysis, we refused chemo treatment. In the view of the doctors, without necessary chemotherapy my mother would have no more than 18 months to live.

My mother is now 82, and no further cancer was found at the six-monthly examinations. The last examination was on 5.7.2006, and after that we dispensed with further check-ups.

Today we are very pleased that we took the right decision (which was very difficult to make at the time).

Nowadays our whole family takes cellular nutrients as precaution.

Yours sincerely
B.B.

Uterine cancer

Dear Dr. Rath

In April 2000 I was diagnosed with uterine carcinoma, which the doctors said was aggressive. Luckily, no lymph nodes had as yet been affected. My womb and ovaries were removed. I was devastated.

During this time a friend told me about Cellular Medicine. I immediately got someone to bring me cellular nutrients at the clinic, and started to take them.

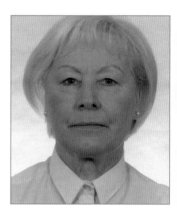

The doctors advised me to have several radiotherapy sessions after the operation, but I refused. I was worried that my bowel or bladder might be harmed. I went back to work just twelve days after the operation – I felt well.

Subsequently, I felt increasingly that cellular nutrients did me a lot of good. I have now been taking them regularly for ten years. All medical tests are clear, and my GP and gynaecologist are very pleased.

Although I am now 71, I am still very lively, youthful and energetic.

I am so grateful that you are there!

With many warm greetings
Your Hildegard Mayer

A world without cancer is at hand!

Prostate cancer

Walter Büttner is a good example of someone who consistently takes responsibility for his own health.

His motto is: Take destiny in your own hands instead of following blindly what others tell you; and this has stood him in good stead through the most difficult periods of his life.

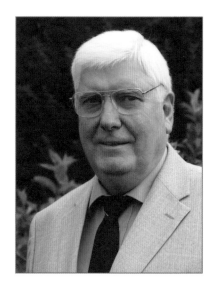

How it all began

How would most of us react if a doctor, in a distanced, professional tone of voice, gave us the shocking diagnosis that we had advanced cancer? Such a statement usually triggers despair in patients, and makes them subject themelves, in blind obedience, to conventional, pharma-oriented medicine. No doubt this was what Walter Büttner's consultant expected when he gave him this diagnosis in 2001. Walter Büttner did not conform to type, however, but replied in his usual calm manner: "So?" Visibly irritated, the doctor referred to the urgency of having surgery within the next few days. Bladder, parts of the small intestine and the prostate were affected, making it essential to remove these organs. Walter Büttner refused, despite the doctor urging this and suggesting that he would otherwise only have three months to live. Unimpressed by this threat, Walter Büttner pursued his own path, repeatedly refused surgery, and today – six years later – feels, in his own words, "healthy and fit as a fiddle".

Finding his own way to health

Resignation and despair don't suit him. Herr Büttner is someone who faces up to critical and difficult situations, and takes his own destiny in hand.

His professional career as a pilot has reinforced his willingness to act decisively and responsibly. Still today – as "unretired pensioner" – his special qualifications as expert on electrohydraulics and aircraft are called upon in the development of ultra-modern simulation technology, both in Germany and abroad. His professional work always required a high degree of responsibility and critical judgement, and naturally this stood him in good stead in relation to his own health.

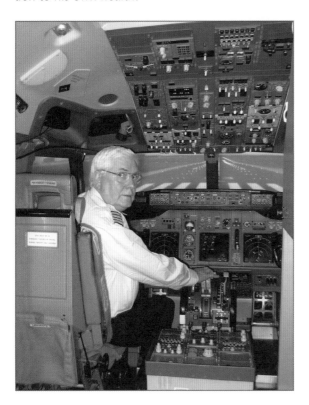

"It was clear to me that the envisaged orthodox procedures – surgery and chemotherapy – were not for me. I was and still am convinced that chemotherapy using substances originally developed as poison gas and combat weapons would harm rather than help me. By lucky chance, I found out about Cellular Medicine."

In fact, this chance had a name, and was the neighbor of one of Walter Büttner's colleagues: Horst Ramershoven, a member of the Health Alliance for many years, met Herrr Büttner shortly after his cancer diagnosis, and had a long talk with him, during which he explained the scientific foundations of Cellular Medicine.

Walter Büttner was convinced by the clarity and logic of Dr. Rath's scientific outlook: "From the outset, Cellular Medicine was a key aspect of my 'self-therapy'. This also included intense scrutiny of myself and my circumstances at the time. Focusing on and resolving professional tensions and conflicts was likewise an important step in healing myself by my own powers."

Appeal to his fellow men

Today, Walter Büttner is a happy and active person, and continues to use cellular nutrients. He is proud and happy that he found the strength to pursue his own path of treatment, and feels the importance of sharing these experiences with others, and encouraging other patients.

We document his appeal on the opposite page.

APPEAL BY WALTER BÜTTNER
TO HIS FELLOW MEN

"I would be very pleased if my own path could act as an example to others.

It is so important to recognize that we are responsible for our own health, and to take this responsibility seriously. Patients should never just blindly obey – however authoritative the person commanding.

Whichever course of action one ultimately decides to pursue, this will at least be the outcome of critical examination, and should also include questioning of the supposed unassailable truths of conventional medicine.

Prostate cancer

Dear Dr. Rath team

My husband, born 1930 and I, born 1938, are well. Thanks for being there!

At the proud age of 81 and 73 we do not need any pharmaceutical drugs, thanks to cellular nutrients.

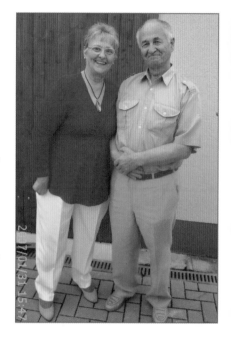

I had stomach cancer and was operated on in 2004. Thank goodness I did not receive any chemotherapy but "only" radiotherapy. Since then I have used cellular nutrients, quickly regaining my strength. So far I am very well, and the cancer has not returned.

My husband was diagnosed with prostate cancer in 2006. He did not accept surgery and also refused the chemotherapy offered to him. His doctors were very annoyed.

He also recovered well thanks to vitamin therapy, and so far has had no further complaints.

We, Family E. Geissler, would like to thank you, and wish the whole team, and Dr. Rath, much continuing success and the best of health.

Thank you!
Your family E + E Geissler

Prostate cancer

Dear Dr. Rath

In March 2003, during a routine check-up, my doctor found my PSA levels were much increased. After this a biopsy was taken, and I was diagnosed with "medium-aggressive cancer".

Around the same time I heard of the positive effects of cellular nutrients on cancer. My urologist recommended radiotherapy, but I decisively rejected this idea.

I used cellular nutrient therapy, which brought the hoped-for outcome. To begin with I included apricot kernels in this regimen.

In March 2004, I had my PSA levels measured for the last time, and they stood at 36. Since then I have had no more such tests.

Over eight years have now passed since the cancer was discovered, and I have absolutely no further complaints.

In the past I also used to suffer from tonsil and gum inflammations. Both these conditions have disappeared too. I don't even get flu any more.

With warm thanks to you and the research team, and many greetings Your Werner K., Münchenstein

Prostate cancer

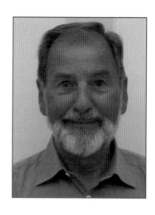

Dear Dr. Rath!

*At the end of 2008 I had breathing prob-
lems and anxiety attacks. The doctor diagnosed cardiac insufficiency (heart weak-
ness) and I was given medication. This
went some way to resolving the problems. I returned to work and went to the
gym regularly. But during a balancing
exercise I fell and broke my fourth cervical vertebra. Surgery had to be
postponed due to the medication I was on. While waiting, I got a severe
infection in the hospital, and the operation had to be postponed until
the infection had subsided and my blood levels were OK again.*

*Questions kept surfacing and I was very doubtful whether everything
was really in order. I was working, working out, and taking my medication; and I went on holiday. Suddenly, as if from nowhere, I had terrible
back pains. Still in Ticino, I went to the emergency department at
Locarno Hospital, and was given painkillers, and advised to get an
examination on my return home to find out the cause of the pain.*

*At the hospital and at my GP's surgery I was told it could be due to
soft tissue rheumatism. I was again given painkillers – but they didn't
really help. Over time I found that passing water was also becoming
painful. I was feeling worse and worse: continually plagued by pain
and losing weight. However, I hoped that each examination I attended would bring a solution.*

*I decided to go to my GP, who knew my whole case history. He did
a blood test and then referred me to a urologist. The urologist did an
ultrasound test and took blood for further tests. He found problems
in the prostate area. I was also referred to Zurich University Hospital
for a bone radio-imaging test.*

The tests showed worrying findings: prostate carcinoma and wide-spread metastasis throughout the bones of the trunk. My subsequent discussion with the urologist did not come up with a satisfactory solution. However, a colleague at work told me about the possibility of natural therapy, and obtained extensive advice for me. I also received information about cellular nutrients. After long discussions with my partner, I decided to pursue the path of Cellular Medicine.

Today I can truly say that I am pain-free: I no longer need painkillers and feel generally lively and well. The check-ups are no longer worrying, and I enjoy my life as a pensioner. PSA levels are measured every six months, and they have fallen from 707 to 268, and then further to 44. The last reading showed a level of 19. A bone radio-imaging test will be done again in the near future, but I am not in the least worried about it: in fact I look forward to the results.

It is important to use cellular nutrients in a rigorous way. There really is a risk that one starts to be a bit lax when one feels better. It is a long-term application that should be strictly adhered to.

My partner supported me in whatever way she could, particularly when it came to strict use of cellular nutrients. Regular contact and discussion with my advisor was also very helpful. I am glad that I went down this route, and therefore suffered no deleterious side effects.

I would like to thank you warmly Dr. Rath for your work, and that of your team. Without your research and tireless commitment, many people might no longer be alive.

With warm greetings
Your Max Baur

Prostate cancer

Dear Dr. Rath

In the spring of 2008, due to ongoing back and stomach complaints, I went to the hospital for a check-up. My troubles were ascribed to gall stones, and these were surgically removed.

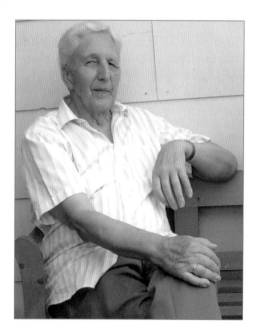

However, this brought no improvement. On the contrary, a few weeks after the gall stone operation, I found myself incapacitated and unable to walk, alongside the pain.

A further examination at the hospital finally brought to light the real cause of my bad state of health. Tumors in the spine were responsible for laming me, and were diagnosed as metastases of a prostate carcinoma.

According to the doctor, immediate surgical intervention was needed on my spine if I was not to face a life confined to the wheelchair.

After surgery and radiotherapy, I and my family were told that I must prepare myself for my imminent end, since the cancer was so advanced.

I refused the chemotherapy I was offered and instead started to take cellular nutrients. As accompaniment to this I drank various herb teas in alternation as indicated in herbalism: green tea, equisetum, rosebay willow herb and stinging nettle. I also took apricot kernels because of their B 17 content.

I am now in a stable condition, almost without pain – as one can see from the attached medical report. I will leave it to others to decide what they think of the verdict by specialists three years ago that I did not have long to live.

I would like to thank the whole Dr. Rath team for their wonderful work, and wish them the very best success for the future.

Warm greetings
Siegfried Obereigner

Prostate cancer

Dear Dr. Rath

About two-and-a-half years ago I was diagnosed with suspected prostate carcinoma. The orthodox medical treatment resulting from this diagnosis – biopsy, surgery, rehab etc. – was not something I wished to embark on.

I therefore decided to use cellular nutrients, alongside another alternative therapy. At the same time I think it is important to take one's own health in hand and to change one's own circumstances and lifestyle accordingly.

All in all, this seems to have been successful so far, for I am feeling well.

Yours sincerely
Dr. W. M.

The latest information on vitamin research in relation to cancer is compiled in these books.

Information on how to order them can be found in the appendix.

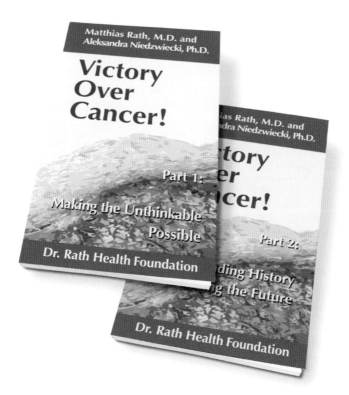

Basic knowledge about leukemia

Leukemia is another common form of cancer.

In chapter 2 of the book "Victory over Cancer!" an explanation is given as to why blood cancer (leukemia) is one of the most common forms of cancer.

In healthy people, white blood corpuscles move through body tissue with the aid of so-called collagen-digesting enzymes. The production of these enzymes is limited in time, and only occurs until the leucocytes have arrived at their destination, e.g. a site of infection.

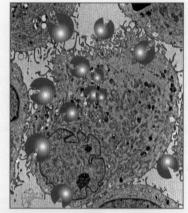

Leukemia cells under a high-resolution electron microscope. The ongoing creation of collagen-digesting enzymes is illustrated by the red "Pac-Men" (see the book "Victory over Cancer!").

When leucocytes become malignant, however, these tissue-dissolving enzymes continue to be incessantly produced.

We can therefore now understand why leukemia is one of the most common types of cancer.

Leukemia

Dear Dr. Rath

Following blood tests in 2002 my doctor gave me the devastating diagnosis of chronic lymphatic leukemia. To begin with I was in despair, believing this would soon prove to be my death sentence. I calmed down a little after discussion with my family and my therapist.

Since I did not wish to undergo chemotherapy if possible, my therapist immediately advised me to take cellular nutrients, which I have been taking every day since then. I also attended a lecture by Dr. Rath at the conference centre in Zurich.

My blood levels (leucocytes and lymphocytes) stayed quite stable; and so far – and ten years have passed now - I have had no need of chemotherapy, and am very pleased and hopeful in consequence.

I am convinced that cellular nutrients have helped me in recent years and I continue to have faith in their health-promoting effect.

Yours sincerely
E.K.

Other types of cancer

Every part of the body can in principle be attacked by cancer. The possible causes of cancer are very diverse and multi-faceted. Key factors, in particular, are cellular nutrient deficiencies, unhealthy diet, psychological pressures, stress, environmental pollution (radiation, car and chemical emissions, pesticides, fungicides etc.), pharmaceutical drugs and suchlike.

Irrespective of the cause and originating organ of cancer, the disseminating mechanism is always the same: the production of collagen-digesting enzymes by cancer cells which thereby create their capacity to spread through the body's tissues.

Cancer of the appendix

Dear Dr. Rath

I have been a faithful user of Cellular Medicine for over ten years. The reason for starting to take cellular nutrients was an appendix operation, following which I was diagnosed with carcinoma of the appendix. I turned down a further, medically recommended colon operation with subsequent chemotherapy, due to negative experiences amongst my friends.

Intake of cellular nutrients led immediately to two health improvements:

- *My gums stopped bleeding, which they had always previously done when I brushed my teeth*

- *I no longer got so many colds and bouts of flu during the winter months*

I am now almost 45, and no further cancer has occurred. The tumor marker CEA shows no pathological findings, and generally I am in very good health.

My mother, M.K., started to take cellular nutrients a few months after I did. She is now 77 and fortunately very sprightly. Her high blood pressure is mostly under good control.

Yours sincerely
H.K.

Medical report for H.K. dated 3.3.1999, confirming the appendix tumor.

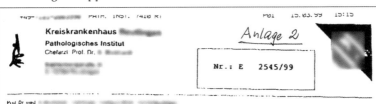

```
+49-                PHIH. INSI. /410 RI              Pol    15.03.99  15:15

     Kreiskrankenhaus
     Pathologisches Institut              Anlage 2
     Chefarzt Prof. Dr.

                                    ┌─────────────────────────┐
                                    │  Nr.: E    2545/99      │
                                    └─────────────────────────┘

Prof Dr med


Herrn Chefarzt                              , 05.03.99 ba/su
Dr. med.
Kreiskrankenhaus                   Name     :   K
Chirurgische Abteilung             Vorname  :   H
                                   geb. am  :
                    KOPIE          Station  :   Chirurgie B

                                   Eingang am: 03.03.99
              Z.Ad. Dr.

Materialbezeichnung:
Appendix.

Klinische Angaben:
Verdacht auf Mukozele. Frage Dignität? Appendixtumor?

Makroskopischer Befund:
Eine 8 cm lange, im Durchmesser bis 1,8 cm messende Appendix. Die
Serosa teilweise mit Fibrin belegt. Das gesamte Appendixlumen ist
von einer grau-weißlichen Gewebemasse ausgefüllt (fr/bö).

Mikroskopischer Befund:
Die histologischen Schnittpräparate zeigen Appendixquerschnitte mit
ausgeweitetem Lumen, in Resten erhaltene Schleimhaut mit
abgeflachten Krypten, hochprismatischen Epithelien und Becherzellen.
Daneben erkennt man eine tubulovillöse Drüsen- und Epithel-
proliferation mit mehrreihigen und mehrschichtigen Epithelanord-
nungen. Die Epithelien zeigen vergrößerte Kerne. Daneben eine
atypische epitheliale Neubildung. Die atypischen Zellen zeigen
Kernhyperchromasie, Kernpolymorphien und Infiltration der Submukosa.

Die Schnittpräparate des Resektionsrandes zeigen Appendixquer-
schnitt mit erhaltener Schleimhaut, hochprismatischen Epithelien,
Becherzellen. Im Schleimhautstroma Lymphozyten, Plasmazellen,
einzelne Granulozyten.

Diagnose:
Hochdifferenziertes Adenokarzinom der Appendix mit Infiltration der
Submukosa im Bereich eines tubulovillösen Adenomes mit hochgradiger
Dysplasie und mäßiggradiger, chronisch-rezidivierender Begleitent-
zündung.

Resektionsrand: Appendixwand, frei von Adenom- oder Karzinomanteile.
```

Diagnosis: Highly differentiated adenocarcinoma of the appendix.

Colon cancer

Dear Dr. Rath

I want to thank you from the bottom of my heart for your research work, and briefly tell you how I am now, and how helpful cellular nutrients have been for me.

In June 2009 I was diagnosed with carcinoma of the rectum. I was to undergo surgery and received chemo and radiotherapy beforehand, to make the carcinoma smaller. In the subsequent operation I was to be given an artificial anus (stoma). This would have severely impaired my quality of life, and I would probably not have been the same person I used to be.

I underwent chemo- and radiotherapy (though reluctantly) but took cellular nutrients and high-dose vitamin C injections to accompany the treatment.

I am convinced that the cellular nutrients a) made the chemotherapy tolerable for me and b) made a major contribution to the final outcome.

In a consultation before the planned operation, the doctor told me that the tumor could no longer be detected. Nevertheless I was due to undergo colostomy surgery the next day. Since the clinical findings showed that none of the tumor could be detected apart from a small remnant, I refused the operation, and instead continued to take cellular nutrients on a daily basis.

At my daughter's urging, after almost two years I underwent another colonoscopy, which found NOTHING at all. The doctor said that I no longer had any cancerous tissue.

If I had allowed myself to be intimidated by the doctors, I would today have a hole in my stomach and a colostomy bag – quite unnecessarily so. I am a hundred percent certain that cellular nutrients helped me a great deal, and I am also endlessly grateful to you! Today, at the age of 69, I still feel very well.

If there were more people like you, more people like me could probably be helped.

During convalescence in a clinic I had to witness that patients are not well-fed, but given food without any real vitamin content that might help them recover. We were continually offered meat and sausage – which in my view is unacceptable.

Particularly in the case of colon cancer one should avoid meat because it easily ferments in the digestive tract.

I am convinced that many people would recover more quickly if they ate fresh, healthy food.

My heartfelt thanks to you. I will continue to use cellular nutrients!

With sunny greetings
M.K.

**Medical reports follow
on the next pages.**

Medical report for M.K. dated 17.7.2009, confirming colon cancer.

Universitätsklinikum

Klinik und Poliklinik für Strahlentherapie
Direktor: Prof. Dr.

Klinik und Poliklinik für Strahlentherapie

1 / 2

An die
Weiterbehandelnden Ärzte
Von
Frau M⬛⬛ K⬛⬛

Ihre Nachricht vom:	Unser Zeichen:	Telefon:	, 17.07.2009
Ihr Zeichen:		Telefax:	
Fallnummer: 0010653189			

Kurzarztbrief

Sehr geehrte Damen und Herren,

wir berichten über die strahlentherapeutische Behandlung von

Patientin:

stationärer Aufenthalt vom 15.07. bis 20.07.09

Diagnose :   Tiefsitzendes Rectum-Ca uT2 N0 M0 G2 PD 05/09

Nebendiagn. :   Z.n. Colon-Ca 2002
                Z.n. Strumektomie

Aktuell: Einleitung einer neoadjuvanten Radiochemotherapie zum
           Sphinctererhalt

Therapie :   Radiatio Becken und Lymphabfluss seit dem 15.07.09 mit simultaner
           Verabreichung von 5-FU in der 1.+ 5. Bestrahlungswoche

Labor :
(15.07.2009)
Klinische Chemie: Natrium: 140 [135 - 145] mmol/l; Kalium: 5.0 [3.5 - 5] mmol/l;
Calcium: 2.3 [2.0 - 2.7] mmol/l; anorg. Phosphat: 1.11 [0.87 - 1.45] mmol/l; Glucose:
90 [82 - 115] mg/dl; glomerul. Filtrationsr. (MDRD): 89 ml/min /1,73qm; Creatinin:
0.7 [0 - 0.95] mg/dl; Harnstoff: 32.1 [10 - 50] mg/dl; Harnsaeure: 3.4 [2.4 - 5.7] mg/dl;
Cholinesterase: 9707 [5320 - 12920] U/l; Gesamt-Bilirubin: 0.3 [0.1 - 1.2] mg/dl;
GOT (ASAT): 18.9 [<= 35] U/l; GPT (ALAT): 21.9 [<= 35] U/l; GGT: 17.0 [<= 40] U/l;
Alk. Phosphatase: 84 [35 - 105] U/l; Lactat Dehydrogenase: 171 [<= 250] U/l;
Gesamt-Eiweiss: 7.2 [6.6 - 8.7] g/dl; Albumin: 4.5 [3.5 - 5.5] g/dl;
Hämatologie: Leukozyten: 5.8 [5 - 10] n*1000/µl; Erythrozyten: 4.52 [4 - 5] n*10E6/µl;
Hämoglobin: 13.3 [12 - 16] g/dl; Hämatokrit: 38.3 [35 - 47] %; MCV: 84.7 [82 - 96] fl;
MCH (HbE): 29.4 [27 - 33] pg; MCHC: 34.7 [32 - 36] g/dl; Thrombozyten: 281 [150 -
450] n*1000/µl;

Anstalt des öffentlichen Rechts

Diagnosis: Deep-seated rectal carcinoma

Two years later the patient had a check-up which found no evidence of the tumor. We have documented these reports on the following pages.

Although the patient asked us to give her initials only when publishing these facts, we have access, of course, to the full medical reports.

Medical report (page 1) for M.K. dated 6.7.2011, confirming that cancer is no longer present.

Tel
Fax

E-mail:
Website:

Dr.med.
Fachärztin für Innere Medizin

Sprechstunden:
Mo-Fr 8.00 - 12.00 Uhr
Mo/Di/Do 15.00 - 17.00 Uhr
und nach Vereinbarung

Dr.med.
Facharzt für Innere Medizin/Gastroenterologie

Internistische Gemeinschaftspraxis
Dr.med.

Frau
M K

06.07.11/

Sehr geehrte Frau K

beiliegend erhalten Sie die aktuellen Untersuchungsergebnisse vom 04.07.11:

Diagnosen:

- Z .n. tief sitzendem Rektumkarzinom (uT2cM0G2);
- Z. n. neo-adjuvanter Radiochemotherapie (keine OP erfolgt);
- Nachsorgeuntersuchung (Restaging);
- Z. n. Colonkarzinom (2002);

Anamnese:
Kommt zur Kontrollkolo bei Z.n. Analpolyp 2009. Therapie: Strahlen und Chemotherapie. Befund war dann "weg". Therapie im ZOM. Vermehrtes Schwitzen. Brennen der Fußsohlen seit der Chemotherapie. Gel. Herzbeschwerden. REHA in (war nichts). 1991 SD-OP. Nimmt SD-Med (Thyroxin 75). Medikamentenanamnese: Thyroxin 75 1-0-0.

Siehe auch Befundberichte der Uniklinik. Offenbar war nach stattgehabter neo-adjuvanter Radiochemotherapie das histologisch-nachgewiesene, tief sitzende Rektumkarzinom, nicht mehr auffindbar gewesen.
Eine weitere proktologische Diagnostik hat die Pat. bis zum aktuellen Zeitpunkt abgelehnt. Stellt sich jetzt zur Verlaufskontrolle – Nachsorge – vor.

Befund:
Größe: 162 cm; Gewicht: 66 kg; Frequenz: 52 /Min. RR bds.: 115/80; BMI: 25 Guter Allgemeinzustand. Haut und Schleimhäute reizfrei. Keine tastbaren Lymphome. Herzaktion regelmäßig. Herztöne rein. Lunge seitengleich belüftet. Abdomen weich, keine tastbaren Resistenzen. Reizfreie Narbe im Unterbauch median und nach Kocher-Schnitt. Nierenlager frei.

Labor:
FT3=4.7 pmol/l; Norm. 3.1- 6.8; FT4=1.6 ng/dl; Norm. 0.9- 1.7 B12=356 pg/ml; Norm. 200- 1000; FOLS=8.5 ng/ml; Norm. 3- 20 Quick=125 %; Norm. 70- 130 INR=0.9 . Leukos=5100 /mm3; Norm. 4000- 10000; HB=13.6 g/dl Norm. 11.7- 15.7; Erys=4.4 10e6/ul; Norm. 3.80- 5.20; HK=38.2 % Norm. 35.0- 47.0; MCV=87 fl; Norm. 81- 100; MCH=30.9 pg Norm. 26.0- 34.0; MCHC=35.6 g/dl; Norm. 31.4- 35.8 Thrombos=292 000/ul; Norm. 150- 400; BZIS=100 mg/dl Norm. 60- 110; HB1C=5.9 %; Norm. < 6.1; HB1CM=41.0 mmol/mol Norm. < 43.2; BILI=0.29 mg/dl; Norm. < 1.00; GOT=23 U/l Norm. < 36; GPT=24 U/l; Norm. < 36; Gamma-GT=20 U/l; Norm. < 39 AP=65 U/l; Norm. 35- 117; Krea=0.73 mg/dl; Norm. < 1.20 TSHLG=1.43 ulE/ml; Norm. 0.35- 4.50.

70

Medical report (page 2) for M.K., dated 6.7.2011, confirming that cancer is no longer present.

Seite 2

M▓▓ K▓▓▓▓

Ruhe-EKG vom 04.07.11:
Bradykarder Sinusrhythmus. Linkstyp.
Inkompletter Rechtsschenkelblock.
Ruhe-EKG Messwerte:

HF	52		P	117 ms		QT	496 ms		ST/II 0.04 mV
QRS	110 ms		PQ	190 ms		QTc	461 ms		
Achse	12 °					QTc-Disp	73 ms.		

Abdomensonographie vom 04.07.11/froh:
Leberstruktur homogen, gering verdichtet. Gallenblase gefüllt, steinfrei. Pankreas gut abgrenzbar, o. B. Nieren o. B., kleine parapelvine Zyste li. Keine pathologischen Darmkokarden. Harnblase gefüllt. Keine Raumforderung im Unterbauch.

Schilddrüsensonographie vom 04.07.11/froh:
Rezidivstruma; insbesondere erheblich vergrößerter li. SD-Lappen, der nach retrosternal reicht. Inhomogene Struktur. Regressive Veränderungen. Inhomogene Perfusion.

Farbdopplerechokardiographie vom 04.07.11/froh:
Herzhöhlen nicht dilatiert, gute linksventrikuläre Kontraktilität, keine intracavitären Massen, keine regionale Dyskinesie, kein Perikarderguß. Klappen morphologisch regelrecht; leichtgradige AI und MI. Hinweis auf eine diastolische Relaxationsstörung.

Zusammenfassung:
Weitere Untersuchungen:
Proktoskopie; Coloskopie, dann auch MR kleines Becken, proktologische Untersuchung in der Uniklinik.

Es wurde aktuell aufgrund der Befunde – kein Anhalt für disseminiertes Tumorgeschehen gesehen.

Mit freundlichen Grüßen

Dr. med. ▓ ▓▓▓▓▓▓

Following the check-up, which included colonoscopy and MRI (magnetic resonance imaging), the medical report concludes with the following summary:

"The findings give no grounds to suspect disseminated* tumor processes."

* Spreading or metastasing

Colon cancer

Dear Dr. Rath

My dear wife fell ill with colon cancer over 14 years ago now. Friends of ours recommended cellular nutrients, and today we are both well.

I decided to take cellular nutrients too, in sympathy – and now I enjoy the same good health as my wife, and am very pleased. We take our 'dose' every day with meals. We also pass on our experiences with this ongoing theme of "health" in our discussion group.

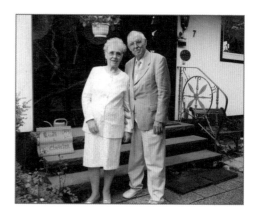

Of course my "statutory" health insurer refused to help with the costs of this provision. They had no wish to acknowledge that we scarcely need to call on their support any more.

It would be a good thing if chemotherapy could be replaced by micronutrients.

With good wishes to the team
Your
Rudi & Christel Kressner

Colon cancer

Dear Dr. Rath

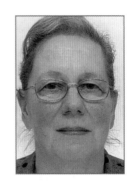

Ten years ago I had aggressive cancer of the colon, and 35 centimetres (about 14 inches) of my intestine were removed.

At that time, unfortunately, I did not yet know anything about the potentially positive effects of cellular nutrients, and although no metastases were present, I allowed myself to be persuaded – I really have to say unfortunately - to have chemotherapy.

After a year-and-a-half a doctor in Salzgitter told me that one might achieve a positive outcome with high-dose vitamins even without chemo. Since then I have sworn by Cellular Medicine, and I am very well indeed! My GP, who does an annual blood test on me, asked me what I was taking since my blood levels were so good – and I told him.

I also try to buy products at the supermarket without E numbers. This is very difficult but it can be done.

My cancer operation was ten years ago, and I feel very well.

And so I thank Dr. Rath and all his helpers for their research work! To the end of my life I will use natural remedies. People don't believe that I am 70 – they think I might be about 55. I never smoked either. Usually I feel strong enough to uproot trees!

Yours sincerely
Your Renate Lai

Colon cancer

Dear Dr. Rath

Cellular nutrients have saved my life.

Firstly, they made my life possible again after a heart attack. The doctors were predicting that I would not live very long – but many years have passed since then. In 1991 I suffered a heart attack. In subsequent years I was given three dilatations and in 1993 even a stent.

Despite a daily dose totaling ten pharmaceutical drugs, my heart attacks did not diminish. After I learned about cellular nutrients in 1994, and from then on took them instead of pharmaceutical drugs, the heart attacks grew fewer. After about half a year they stopped altogether, and my heart capacity got better and better.

Secondly, after my colon cancer, a malignant tumor, cellular nutrients helped me regain my health. I received this diagnosis in 2009. The tumor was surgically removed along with 36 centimetres (about 14 inches) of intestine and a stoma inserted. At the time the doctors were unable to understand that there were no metastases. The anesthesiologist even asked me whether I was taking cellular nutrients, since this type of cancer is usually very aggressive.

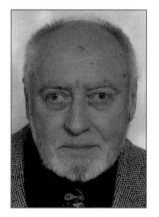

Fortunately, after about a year, it was possible to reverse the stoma procedure again.

For several years now I have been completely free of cancer through using cellular nutrients. I am now 78 and feel very well. I owe all this to you Dr. Rath, and I thank you most warmly for it.

Yours sincerely
Hermann Lehnert

Colon cancer

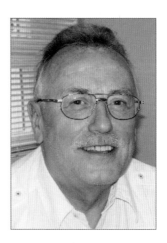

Dear ladies and gentlemen

In 1999 I fell ill with colon cancer and was operated on in August of the same year. Following subsequent check-ups in 2001 it was discovered that a metastasis had migrated to my lungs during the operation and had grown into a new tumor there. During further surgery the top left lobe of my lung was removed.

After surviving the operation, a good friend suggested I find out about Cellular Medicine online. I was very interested and, after an advisory session, started to take cellular nutrients.

After a couple of months I had the feeling that my general state of health had improved, and this was confirmed in subsequent check-ups.

Colonoscopy and MRI scans resulted in no pathological findings. My GP also told me that my test results were on a par with those of a healthy person, and that I could be considered cured.

Since then I still continue to take cellular nutrients, and feel very well.

Yours sincerely
B. Rohrbach

Colon cancer

Dear Dr. Rath team

In 2000 I received a devastating diagnosis: aggressive colon cancer.
I had to undergo an operation immediately. A year later a liver metastasis was discovered, which likewise had to be operated on.

I started searching for ways of supporting my body with natural substances.

In 2002 someone recommended Cellular Medicine to me, and I found it convincing.

I placed my trust in cellular nutrients and am sure that they helped me to recover my health. Naturally I also changed my diet.

Happily I can report that I am well. To ensure things stay like that I will carry on in the same way.

At every opportunity I recommend cellular nutrients and tell people about my good state of health. I am so convinced that I now work in the Health Alliance and am glad to help others by providing education and information.

Yours sincerely
Lore Krenedics

Colon cancer

Dear Dr. Rath MD

In 2002 and 2003, I had to undergo two colon cancer operations, with stoma. The last reversal of the procedure took place in August 2003.

Since then I have been taking cellular nutrients on a daily basis, and find I have no complications affecting my digestion, let alone any recurrence of the colon cancer.

I attribute this fact to regular use of cellular nutrients.

Yours sincerely
K.-R. T.

Bladder cancer

Dear Dr. Rath

In August of this year I will be 75. When I was about 60 (1996) my GP found blood in my urine.

Subsequently a urologist did an endoscopy of my urinary tract, and diagnosed bladder carcinoma. In the following eight years I underwent eight operations to remove the tumor. Each year it grew back again with continuous regularity.

Until… yes, until, due to a misdiagnosis by the urologist who had treated me so far, I changed doctors. At a check-up he had failed to notice the presence of a tumor in the bladder.

After an endoscopy, the new urologist I had chosen found a tumor in the front of the bladder, and explained the misdiagnosis by the fact that until then the focus had been only on the rear bladder wall, so that the tumor was not noticed.

At the hospital – also a new one that I chose! – I was operated on twice in five weeks, since the danger of bladder perforation meant that just one operation was not possible. Subsequently, at the rec-ommendation of the chief urology consultant, treatment with Metamycin was started in order to prevent the tumor from grow-ing back again. This was a kind of localized chemotherapy, since the substance was injected straight into the bladder and had to stay there for several hours.

Seven years have passed since then without any detectable recur-rence of the bladder tumor. My bladder was checked a total of 35 times by a urologist, using endoscopy. By nature I am rather scep-tical, and my anxiety after every check-up remains, until the good results come through.

But now to you, Dr. Rath! Around the time of my last bladder operation an acquaintance told me of the positive effects of cellular nutrients. Since then I have been taking them regularly, and am pretty sure that they prevented a recurrence of the tumor by strengthening my immune system.

For the sake of completeness I would also mention that my health lifestyle also includes other factors such as regular exercise, physical activity, healthy diet, enough fluids, and almost no alcohol. I am also a non-smoker!

I would ask you to use a pseudonym when publishing this letter.

Yours sincerely
G.B.

Sinus cancer

Dear Dr. Rath

Below I will give you a short account of how I came to cellular nutrients.

In 1998 I had angina. I was unable to walk even 30 metres without having to rest. My next stop was my GP. What did he prescribe? Betablockers.

My professional work had brought me into contact with a professor (of medicine). We often had conversations about illness. At each conversation he told me, "Let me warn you against chemo." This comment encouraged me to look for natural remedies on the market. By chance I obtained your address. Within the first four weeks, cellular nutrients improved my health. After three months I was problem-free.

In 2007 I had to have surgery on a sinus tumor. After the operation, 30 sessions of radiotherapy were prescribed, which I refused. In the meantime I had had good experience with cellular nutrients. In addition I received vitamin C infusions from a naturopath.

I am well, and the illness never returned.

Yours sincerely
Otto Hölzemann

Indications: Condition following nasal sinus exploration on both sides with rhinoplasty following histologically ascertained adenocarcinoma of the right nostril and nasal sinus.

Medical report for Otto Hölzemann dated 10.12.2007, confirming sinus cancer

Universitätsklinikum
Anstalt des öffentlichen Rechts

Klinik und Poliklinik für Hals-, Nasen- u. Ohrenheilkunde
Direktor: Univ.- Prof. Dr. med.

Stat.: O3

Datum: 10.12.2007/So

Name: Hölzemann   Vorname: Otto

geb.: 04.03.1929

O P E R A T I O N S B E R I C H T

Operateur: OA Dr. med.
Dr. med.

Anästhesist: OA Dr. med.

Assistenten:

OP-Pflegepersonal:

Indikationen:
Zustand nach Nasennebenhöhlenexploration beidseits mit Septumplastik bei bereits histologisch gesichertem Adenokarzinom der rechten Nasenhaupt- und Nasennebenhöhle am 21.11.2007

Ausgeführte Operation: Radikale Pansinusoperation rechts mit transantralem Zugang rechts

Operationsbericht:
Zunächst Entfernung der Doyle-Splints beidseits. Anschließend Inspektion der Nasenhaupthöhle beidseits. Conchektomie sowohl der unteren als auch der mittleren Nasenmuschel rechts. Es findet sich noch tumoröses Gewebe im Bereich der hinteren Muschelenden Übergang zum Nasopharynx. Dieser Bereich wird sukzessiv von Tumormassen befreit. Die Septumschleimhaut in Area IV erscheint hyperplastisch. Sicherheitshalber Entnahme einer PE aus diesem Bereich und Einsenden zur Schnellschnittuntersuchung. Diese ergibt soweit keinen Anhalt für Malignität. Ausräumen des gesamten Siebbeinzellsystems und der Keilbeinhöhle unter Darstellung der Schädelbasis. Dabei kommt die Dura im Übergang zwischen cranialem Septum und Schädelbasis frei zu liegen. Liquor tritt soweit nicht heraus. Im Bereich der Lamina papyracea ebenfalls Entfernen von Tumormassen, wobei ein Teil der Lamina papyracea mit entfernt wird. Dadurch kommt es zum Fettprolaps. Großzügiges Eröffnen des Zugangs zur Kieferhöhle. Hierüber lässt sich massenhaft tumoröses Gewebe entfernen. Es gelingt nicht das Tumorgewebe komplett zu entfernen, so dass ein zusätzlicher transantraler Zugang rechts zur Kieferhöhle erforderlich ist. Darstellen des vestibulum oris. Einschneiden oberhalb der Zahnleiste auf den Os maxillare rechts. Abschieben der Gesichtsweichteile von der Vorderwand des Os maxillare mittels Raspatorium ohne Tangierung des N. infraorbitalis. Entfernung der Kieferhöhlenvorderwand mittels Rosenbohrer. Danach lässt sich eine optimale Übersicht über die Kieferhöhle gewinnen. Entfernung des Resttumorgewebe. Im Bereich des Orbitabodens kommt dabei ein kleiner Frakturspalt zur Geltung, worüber wenig orbitales Fettgewebe in die Kieferhöhle tropfenförmig sich vorschiebt. Dieser Bereich wird nicht weiter tangiert. Zum Abschluss noch mal endoskopische Kontrolle der gesamten Nasennebenhöhle rechts mittels 30° und 70° Optik. Insgesamt konnte soweit mikroskopisch als auch endoskopisch der Tumor komplett entfernt werden. Abdecken der freiliegenden Dura mittels Tissue Dura Fibrinkleber

Medical report follows on the following pages

Medical report for Otto Hölzemann dated 26.4.2011, confirming that cancer is no longer present.

Printed information   Seite 1 von 1

Report HÖLZEMANN, OTTO   MRT VON SCHAEDEL UND HALS ▓▓▓▓▓▓ ▓▓
Report:
Z. n. Adenokarzinom NNH, ED 11/07; Beschwerdezunahme
Rezidiv? Spiegelbefund? (???)

MRT des Gesichtsschädel/Halses vom 26.04.2011:

Zum Vergleich CT-Schädel-Voruntersuchung vom 07.04.2010.

Befund:
Im Vergleich zur Voruntersuchung bei nun anderer Modalität in der rechten Kieferhöhle 19 mm x 12 mm große glatt berandete, in T1 und T2 überwiegend hyperintense Raumforderung (ima 4/27). Kein Nachweis einer malignitätsverdächtigen Raumforderung in der NHH und den NNH. Z. n. Tumorexstirpation rechts mit Resektion der medialen Orbitawand/des Orbitabodens, partieller Resektion der Ethmoidalzellen sowie der Nasenmuscheln rechts mit anschließender Defektdeckung wie vorbestehend.
Unauffällige Darstellung von Larynx und Pharynx.
Kein Nachweis einer intracraniellen Raumforderung.
Kein Nachweis pathologisch vergrößerter Lymphknoten.
Kein Nachweis einer malignitätsverdächtigen knöchernen Veränderung.
Kein Nachweis einer Raumforderung in den mitabgebildeten thorakalen Abschnitten.

Beurteilung:
1. Kein Anhalt für ein Lokalrezidiv nach Resektion des vormaligen Adenokarzinoms.
2. A. e. Mucoidzyste rechte Kieferhöhle.
3. Kein Nachweis pathologisch vergrößerter Lymphknoten.

Req. Physician-Service: Station HNOP
Patient: Hölzemann Otto ▓▓▓▓▓▓
Date of Exam: 26.04.2011 10:42
Accession Nr.: 1771204
Report Author: Dr. med. ▓▓▓▓▓ ▓▓▓▓
Report Approver: OÄ Dr. med. ▓▓▓▓ ▓▓▓▓▓
Rep. Creation Date: 26.04.2011 13:45

Findings (extract):

No evidence of intracranial tumor mass.
No evidence of pathologically enlarged lymph nodes.

No evidence of bone changes indicative of malignancy.

No evidence of tumor mass in the thoracic sections
included in imaging.

Thyroid cancer

Dear Dr. Rath

First of all I would like to thank you for your outstanding work and commitment!

I have been using cellular nutrients for the past eleven years with complete satisfaction. Back then I was diagnosed with thyroid cancer, and had to undergo two operations which filled me with anxiety and uncertainty. I was devastated. Then a friend told me about you.

I followed the principles of Cellular Medicine and soon felt better.

At the clinic I met a couple of women who had also been using cellular nutrients with great satisfaction. I also told the professor about this, and he said this was a good thing and I should continue. Now I felt absolutely sure.

Almost eleven years have passed since then. The 10-year checkup is now behind me. My body is free of disease, and thanks to cellular medical treatment the illness never recurred.

I wish you much continued success with your research, and hope that you will be able to go on helping many more like me.

With warm thanks
Your Antonia Pail

Kidney cancer

Dear Dr. Rath

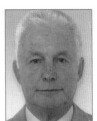

I have been a cancer patient since 1993 (metastasizing kidney carcinoma). In October 1993 my left kidney was surgically removed, and then in 2003/04, metastases in the right buttock, left thigh and both lungs. After surgery in December 2003, chemotherapy followed in January/February 2004, but this had to be stopped again after two sessions since three further operations were due.

After this I decided to pursue biological cancer therapy based on cellular nutrients. I gathered extensive information about scientific findings relating to the use of cellular nutrients, and reports by those who had used them. I also completed the basic and further training course at the Dr. Rath Health Alliance, and took an active part in many Health Alliance events.

"Biological cancer therapy" was accompanied by regular radiological tests and blood analyses. These confirmed that my health was stable, thus demonstrating how effective my chosen therapy was. At 75 I now feel in a good state.

I am convinced that cellular nutrients, which I have been taking since April 2004, have had a very positive effect on my overall health.

This is why I am a member of the Dr. Rath Health Alliance, and have also passed my experiences on to others, to good effect.

Yours sincerely
Professor Dr. Manfred Reiss

Lymph gland cancer

Dear friends

I would like to tell you about my wife's state of health:

My wife, Marthe Robert (born 1929) was diagnosed with lymph gland cancer in 2002.

As usual (!) chemotherapy was prescribed. However, this affected her so badly that it was stopped after six treatments (rather than eight). This led to a week in hospital with acute shingles.

It seemed the doctors had no other choice than to prescribe radiotherapy. But when we heard that her whole body was to be exposed to this treatment, which would, at the same time, have led to nerve damage, we decided against it. This was also because we had started to take cellular nutrients at this time, at the recommendation of a Dr. Rath Health Alliance advisor.

Two years later she had a relapse. We found another doctor who seemingly gave "gentler" chemotherapy in his practice. This time my wife coped well with the treatment (without losing her hair).

The doctor later told us that in the case of recurrence there was usually only a 25 percent chance of recovery. However, already during treatment, and also at its conclusion, the results were good. Clearly the cellular nutrients had helped bring about a cure. After five years (with annual medical check-ups) my wife was at last well again.

Now seven years have passed and – by God's help too – we are in the best of health, for which we are very grateful.

Yours sincerely
A. and M. Robert

Lung cancer

My name is Werner Pilniok

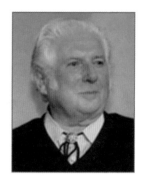

In September 1999, during a routine x-ray, I was diagnosed with a fast-growing lung tumor. According to the doctor, a pneumologist, this tumor measured 1.5 x 1 centimetres (0.6 x 0.4 inches). I underwent a series of further tests, after which the doctors recommended surgical intervention and removal of the whole lung section where the tumor was situated.

But since I suffered from heart disease, an operation would have been very risky for me. I therefore started to look around for alternatives. I read about the research by Dr. Rath, who was studying the role of cellular nutrients in natural treatment of cancer and other illnesses.

I decided to cancel the planned operation and to give micronutrients a chance. From October 1999 on, I supplemented my diet with a large quantity of micronutrients.

On 3 April 2000 I had a CT scan which showed that the tumor found six months before had disappeared! My doctors couldn't believe it. They asked me to come back again a few days later, since clearly they thought the scanning machine must be faulty. But the new scan showed the same result – the tumor was no longer there.

This was more than a decade ago. In 2011 I celebrated my 80th birthday in good health. Thanks to micronutrients I hope to live many more years still.

Werner Pilniok

Top: scan of Herr Pilniok's lung at the time
that lung cancer was diagnosed.

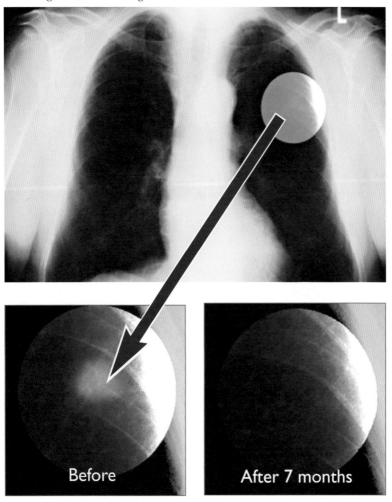

Bottom left: enlarged section of the lung scan.
Bottom right: scan of the same portion of lung after seven months
of taking cellular nutrients.

Lung cancer

Dear Dr. Rath

Six years ago, in May 2005, I was found to have lung cancer, and my top right lung lobe was surgically removed. Since then I have been taking cellular nutrients. My state of health is very good, and above all stable. I am not taking any additional medicines. The lung specialist whom I go to see regularly is amazed at my recovery.

My wife is also taking cellular nutrients and, since she began, has no longer suffered from heartburn and stomach pain. Her digestion is in order again. My daughter also swears by cellular nutrients, which she has been taking for a year now. Her allergy is much better and she no longer gets colds although she is in daily contact with patients.

In conclusion we can say that we are all in much better health. I hope that this continues.

Yours sincerely
Rudolf Schernhammer

Cancer of the parotid gland

Dear Dr. Rath

My name is Bozana Schneeberger. I live in the Tyrol but was born in Croatia.

In 2007, I was found to have severe cancer of the parotid gland. My world fell apart.

I was first operated on shortly after the diagnosis, in 2007. The surgery lasted for eight hours. Afterwards the surgeon told me that the tumor was interwoven with the facial nerve, and that he was unable to help any further. The tumor was 3.6 centimetres (about 1.4 inches) in size!

A week after the operation, my condition had further deteriorated. An MRI scan showed that the tumor had spread to an artery.

On 12.6.2007 a friend brought me cellular nutrients and I took a triple dose every day since my only hope was that it would help me, that it must help me, as it had helped others.

On 18.7.2007, shortly before my second operation, another MRI scan was taken. On the afternoon of the same day, the Professor told me that my tumor had almost completely vanished: only a small dot could now be seen.

I knew this would be so, and I immediately told him about cellular nutrients, which I always had beside my bed. The doctor was from Germany and said he knew who Dr. Rath was and that I should carry on taking them. After surgery my medical report stated: 'Tumor-free'. At the time I said that I would like to meet Dr. Rath in person. On 18.2.2008, therefore, I got into my car and drove to Holland. I just wanted to have a picture of Dr. Rath, and to promise him that I will help others and tell them what cellular nutrients did for me, and how they work in the body.

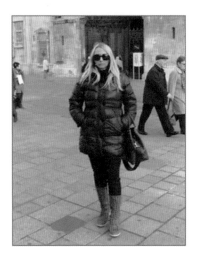

I am very glad to have avoided chemotherapy – which does no good since it is just big business. I would like to advise everyone not to wait until cancer strikes but to prevent it with cellular nutrients!

Finally I would like to thank you Dr. Rath for giving me back my life so that I can tell my story to others.

Your Bozana Schneeberger

Non-Hodgkin lymphoma

Dear Dr. Rath

In 2005 my husband received the devastating diagnosis of cancer. He was operated on, since the doctors thought he was suffering from colon cancer. However this was not the case, and it later turned out that it was very malignant non-Hodgkin lymphoma.

My husband started with chemotherapy, but stopped it again after a while.

At the recommendation of my brother-in-law, Gabriel Lommer, we are now taking cellular nutrients.

In the meantime my husband is very well again.

I myself was thankfully never seriously ill, though my husband's cancer was a very stressful period for me. I had high cholesterol levels, but got a grip on them thanks to cellular nutrients.

We feel fit and energetic and like working in our large garden. I myself am still working part-time in catering, after working in a bank for 35 years. I also often look after our three grandchildren!

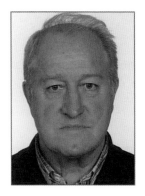 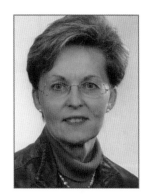

The information you provide, such as Rath International and your Health letters, frequently contain valuable tips. In the meantime we have also been able to get a few friends very interested in Cellular Medicine.

Our day starts with cellular nutrients, and we are pleased that we can cope so well with our active workload.

*Yours sincerely
The Schütt family*

Non-Hodgkin lymphoma

Dear ladies and gentlemen

On 1.4.2008 I was diagnosed with a tumor in the upper abdomen measuring 5.6 x 3.8 centimetres (about 2.2 x 1.5 inches), and a second tumor of 2 centimetres (about 3/4 inch) in diameter (CT scan). After undergoing all tests I was told that this was a grade 2 non-Hodgkin lymphoma of low malignancy.

I rejected the route of orthodox medicine involving surgery, chemo or radiotherapy in order to pursue my own path. I got information about cellular nutrients and started to take them at the end of July 2008.

Alongside this I used homeopathic remedies and was given vitamin C infusions. I did this for a year, and continued working full-time in absolute certainty of what I was doing.

On 6.10.2008 an MRI scan showed that the lymphoma had reduced in size to 4.5 x 2.3 centimetres (1.7 x 0.9 inches), and the second tumor to a diameter of 1.6 centimetres (0.6 inch). In other words, my decision had been right.

On 24.11.2010, the large tumor measured only 2.2 x 1.8 x 2.1 centimetres (3/4 x 0.7 x 3/4 inch), and the small one could no longer be detected at all.

My goal is clear and I will carry on. I feel very well, and am happy that I took this route.

Yours sincerely
Edeltraud Schwörer

Medical report for Edeltraud Schwörer on 14.4.2008, showing a tumor size of 5.6 x 3.8 cm.

Radiologie

Fachärzte für Radiologie
Dr. med.
Dr. med.
Dr. med.
Dr. med.

Dr. med.
Dr. med

Telefon
Telefax
Computertomographie
Kernspintomographie

Herrn
Dr. med.

14.04.2008/

Sehr geehrter Herr Kollege

vielen Dank für die freundliche Überweisung Ihrer Patientin

Edeltraud Schwörer, geb.

CT Abdomen vom 10.04.2008

Fragestellung:
V. a. Raumforderung Pankreas.

Methode:
Wir untersuchten nach Applikation von KM I. v. mit Mehrzeilen-CT-Technik.

Zusammenfassender Befund und Beurteilung:
Linksseitig findet sich ab Höhe des Nierenhilus links retroperitoneal paraaortal eine 5.6 x 3.8 cm messende Raumforderung, die mit einer gleichartigen Gewebsstruktur zusammenhängt, die weiter caudal nach rechts dorsal der Aorta, ventral der Wirbelsäule die Mittellinie überschreitet. Diese Raumforderung steht nicht mit dem Pankreas zusammen, das unauffällig abgebildet ist. Im Oberbauch fällt im übrigen eine blande, 1 cm messende Nierenzyste am cranialen Bereich der Niere auf.
Keine Leberfiliae. Caudal des größeren Tumors liegt links paraaortal ein knapp 2 cm messender, metastasenverdächtiger Lymphknoten vor, im kleinen Becken keine Auffälligkeiten.
Zusammenfassend Nachweis eines NPL-verdächtigen retroperitonealen Tumors links im Ober-/ ittelbauch, neben dem Vorliegen eines Lymphoms käme auch ein sarkomatöser Prozeß in Frage.

Filme zum Verbleib wurden mitgegeben.

**Summary of findings and assessment (excerpt):
Tumor mass on the left side, at kidney hilum level, measuring 5.6 x 3.8 cm.**

In summary, evidence of an retroperitoneal tumor suspected of being an NPL*

* Neoplasm = cancer

Edeltraud Schwörer: At the check-up 4 1/2 years later,
the tumor only measured 4.5 x 2.3 cm (1.7 x 0.9 inches), and had
therefore diminished considerably in size.

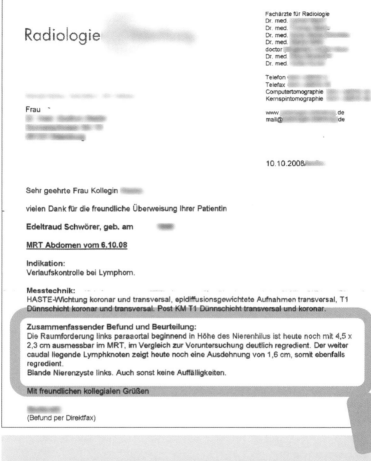

Radiologie

Fachärzte für Radiologie
Dr. med.
Dr. med.
Dr. med.
Dr. med.
doctor
Dr. med
Dr. med.

Telefon
Telefax
Computertomographie
Kernspintomographie

Frau

www .de
mail@ .de

10.10.2008/

Sehr geehrte Frau Kollegin

vielen Dank für die freundliche Überweisung Ihrer Patientin

Edeltraud Schwörer, geb. am

MRT Abdomen vom 6.10.08

Indikation:
Verlaufskontrolle bei Lymphom.

Messtechnik:
HASTE-Wichtung koronar und transversal, epidiffusionsgewichtete Aufnahmen transversal, T1
Dünnschicht koronar und transversal. Post KM T1 Dünnschicht transversal und koronar.

Zusammenfassender Befund und Beurteilung:
Die Raumforderung links paraaortal beginnend in Höhe des Nierenhilus ist heute noch mit 4,5 x
2,3 cm ausmessbar im MRT, im Vergleich zur Voruntersuchung deutlich regredient. Der weiter
caudal liegende Lymphknoten zeigt heute noch eine Ausdehnung von 1,6 cm, somit ebenfalls
regredient.
Blande Nierenzyste links. Auch sonst keine Auffälligkeiten.

Mit freundlichen kollegialen Grüßen

(Befund per Direktfax)

Summary of findings and assessment: The para-aortal tumor mass on
the left side, at the level of the kidney hilum, now measures 4.5 x 2.3
cm in the MRI scan, and is clearly regressing compared to the previ-
ous examination. The more caudally situated lymph node now measures 1.6 cm and is thus likewise regressing. Kidney cyst left, of no
concern. No other detectable symptoms.

Edeltraud Schwörer: At the check-up three years later, the tumor had shrunk still further and now measured 2.3 x 2.1 x 1.8 cm.

Radiologie

Radiologie
Dr. med. ████
Dr. med. ████
Dr. med. ████
Dr. med. ████
████
Dr. med. ████
Dr. med. ████
Fachärzte für Radiologie

Nuklearmedizin
Dr. med. ████
Facharzt für Nuklearmedizin u. Radiologie

Radiologie ████

Frau
Edeltraud Schwörer

Telefon ████
Telefax ████
Computertomographie ████
Kernspintomographie ████
www. ████ .de
mail @ ████ .de

26.11.2010/ NIE/R

Sehr geehrte Frau Schwörer,

nachfolgend berichten wir über Ihre Untersuchung vom 24.11.10.

<u>Sonographie Abdomen</u>

Klinische Angaben:
Verlaufskontrolle bei Z. n. Lymphom.

Befund und Beurteilung:
Der vorbekannte Lymphknoten unterhalb der linken Nierenvene von ehemals 4.3 x 2.2 x 2.5 cm (Juni d. J.) auf nun 2.3 x 2.1 x 1.8 cm Größe verkleinert.
Oberbauchorgane und Unterbauch regelrecht. Keine neu aufgetretenen Lymphome auch retroperitoneal und entlang der Beckenstrombahn.

Die Bilder und ein Kurzbefund wurden mitgegeben.

Mit freundlichen Grüßen

Dr. ████

Nachrichtlich: Dr. med. ████

Acknowledgements

Heartfelt thanks to all patients who had the courage to share their experiences in this book.

Our special recognition goes to all patients, young and old, who had no opportunity to fight their illness, and who might have had a chance if they had not wasted so much time in the dead-end of conventional medicine.

Our thanks to Dr. Matthias Rath, Dr. Aleksandra Niedzwiecki, director of our research institute, and our whole research team, who have corroborated this medical breakthrough with creativity and persistence. Our special thanks goes to Dr. Waheed Roomi, head of our cancer research department, who has been undertaking and supervising these important experiments for over a decade. We also thank Dr. Shrirang Netke, Dr. Vadim Ivanov, Dr. Raxit Jariwalla, Nusrath Roomi and Tatiana Kalinovsky for helping this innovative research to progress and develop.

A very special thanks to Manja Heidemann for her work in compiling this book, and to Renate Ottofrickenstein and Bernd-Ulrich Rüller for their assistance. We thank Jörg Wortmann for his work on the layout and Anke Wartenberg for proofreading.

Special thanks to the many thousands of members of our international Health Alliance, which has been supporting our research work for over a decade. Without them this breakthrough would not have been possible.

Finally we would like to thank all those whose skepticism and resistance has provided an invaluable stimulus to our own motivation.

Dr. Rath Health Foundation

Appendix

Publication of our findings

PROSTATE CANCER
In Vivo Antitumor Effect of Ascorbic Acid, Lysine, Proline and Green Tea Extract on Human Prostate PC-3 Xenografts in Nude Mice: Evaluation of Tumor Growth and Immunohistochemistry. M.W. Roomi, V. Ivanov, T. Kalinovsky, A. Niedzwiecki, M. Rath. *In Vivo , 2005, 19(1), 179-184.*

Antitumor Effect of Ascorbic Acid, Lysine, Proline, Arginine and Epigallocatechin Gallate in Prostate Cancer Cell Lines PC-3, NCaP, and DU145. M.W. Roomi, V. Ivanov, T. Kalinovsky, A. Niedzwiecki, M. Rath
Research Communications in Molecular Pathology and Pharmacology, 2004, 115:1-6

TESTICULAR CANCER
Inhibitory Effects of a Nutrient Mixture on Human Testicular Cancer cell Line NT 2/DT Matrigel Invasion and MMP Activity. M.W. Roomi, V. Ivanov, T. Kalinovsky, A. Niedzwiecki, M. Rath. *Medical Oncology 2007 24(2): 183-188*

BREAST CANCER
In Vitro and In Vivo Antitumorigenic Activity of a Mixture of Lysine, Proline, Ascorbic Acid and Green Tea Extract on Human Breast Cancer Lines MDA MB-231 and MCF-7. M.W. Roomi, V. Ivanov, T. Kalinovsky, A. Niedzwiecki, M. Rath *Medical Oncology 2005, 22(2) 129-38*

Modulation of N-Methyl –N-Nitrosourea-Induced Mammary Tumors in Sprague-Dawley Rats by Combination of Lysine, Proline, Arginine, Ascorbic Acid and Green Tea Extract. M.W. Roomi, N.W. Roomi, V. Ivanov, T. Kalinovsky, A. Niedzwiecki, M. Rath. Breast Cancer Research, 2005, 7:R291-R295

A combination of green tea extract, specific nutrient mixture and quercetin: An effective intervention treatment for the regression of N-Methyl –N-Nitrosourea (MNU)-Induced mammary tumors in Wistar rats. Anup Kale, Sonia Gawande, Swati Kotwal, Shrirang Netke, M.W. Roomi, V. Ivanov, A. Niedzwiecki, M. Rath *Oncology Letters, 2010, 1:313-317*

CERVICAL CANCER

Suppression of Human Cervical Cancer Cell Lines Hela and oTc2 4510 MMP Expression and Matrigel Invasion by a Mixture of Lysine, Proline, Ascorbic Acid, and Green Tea Extract. M.W. Roomi, V. Ivanov, T. Kalinovsky, A. Niedzwiecki, M.Rath *International Journal of Gynecological Cancer 2006; 16:1241-1247*

OVARIAN CANCER

In vitro modulation of MMP-2 and MMP-9 in human cervical and ovarian cancer cell lines by cytokines, inducers and inhibitors. M.W. Roomi, J.C. Monterrey, T. Kalinovsky, M. Rath, A. Niedzwiecki. *Oncology Reports 2010; 23(3):605-614*

Inhibition of MMP-2 Secretion and Invasion by Human Ovarian Cancer Cell Line SKOV-3 with lysine, proline, arginine, ascorbic acid, and Green Tea Extract. M.W. Roomi, V. Ivanov, T. Kalinovsky, A. Niedzwiecki, M. Rath *Journal of Obstetrics and Gynaecology Research 2006; 32(2): 148-154*

COLON CANCER

In Vivo Antitumor Effect of Ascorbic Acid, Lysine, Proline and Green Tea Extract on Human Colon Cancer Cell HCT 116 Xenografts in Nude Mice: Evaluation of Tumor Growth and Immunohistochemistry. M.W. Roomi, V. Ivanov, T. Kalinovsky, A. Niedzwiecki, M. Rath. *Oncology Reports, 2005, 12 (3), 421-425*

Synergistic Effect of Combination of Lysine, Proline, Arginine, Ascorbic Acid and Epigallocatechin Gallate on Colon Cancer Cell Line HCT 116. M.W. Roomi, V. Ivanov, T. Kalinovsky, A. Niedzwiecki, M. Rath *Journal of the American Nutraceutical Association, 2004, 7 (2): 40-43*

BONE CANCER

Naturally Produced Extracellular Matrix Inhibits Growth Rate and Invasiveness of Human Osteosarcoma Cancer Cells. V. Ivanov, S. Ivanova, M.W. Roomi, T. Kalinovsky, A. Niedzwiecki, M. Rath. *Medical Oncology 2007; 24(2): 209-217*

Effect of Ascorbic Acid, Lysine, Proline and Green Tea Extract on Human Osteosarcoma Cell Line MNNG-HOS Xenografts in Nude Mice: Evaluation of Tumor Growth and Immunohistochemistry. M.W. Roomi, V. Ivanov, T. Kalinovsky, A. Niedzwiecki, M. Rath. *Medical Oncology 2006; 23(3): 411-417*

Antitumor Effect of Nutrient Synergy on Human Osteosarcoma Cells U2OS, MNNGHOS, and Ewing's Sarcoma SK-ES.1. M.W. Roomi, V. Ivanov, T. Kalinovsky, A. Niedzwiecki, M. Rath. *Oncology Reports, 2005, 13(2), 253-257*

In Vivo and In Vitro Antitumor Effect of Nutrient Synergy on Human Osteosarcoma Cell Line MNNG-HOS. M.W. Roomi, V. Ivanov, T. Kalinovsky, A. Niedzwiecki, M. Rath. *Annals of Cancer Research and Therapy, 2004, 12: 137-148*

PANCREATIC CANCER

Antitumor Effect of a Combination of Lysine, Proline, Arginine, Ascorbic Acid, and Green Tea Extract on Pancreatic Cancer Cell Line MIA PaCa-2. M.W. Roomi, V. Ivanov, T. Kalinovsky, A. Niedzwiecki, M. Rath
International Journal of Gastrointestinal Cancer 2005, 35 (2), 97-102

FIBROSARCOMA

In Vivo and in Vitro Antitumor Effect of Ascorbic Acid, Lysine, Proline, Arginine, and Green Tea Extract on Human Fibrosarcoma Cells HT-1080. M.W. Roomi, V. Ivanov, T. Kalinovsky, A. Niedzwiecki, M. Rath
Medical Oncology 2006; 23(1): 105-112

Synergistic Antitumor Effect of Ascorbic Acid, Lysine, Proline, and Epigallocatechin Gallate on Human Fibrosarcoma Cells HT-1080. M.W. Roomi, V. Ivanov, T. Kalinovsky, A. Niedzwiecki, M. Rath
Annals of Cancer Research and Therapy, 2004 12:148-157

KIDNEY AND BLADDER CANCER

Pleiotropic effects of a micronutrient mixture on critical parameters of bladder cancer. M.W. Roomi, T. Kalinovsky, A. Niedzwiecki, M. Rath. In Bladder Cancer: Etymology, *Diagnosis and Treatments, edited by William Nilsson, Nova Science Publishers, Inc, 2010.*

Antitumor Effect of Ascorbic Acid, Lysine, Proline, Arginine, and Green Tea Extract on Bladder Cancer Cell Line T-24. M.W. Roomi, V. Ivanov, T. Kalinovsky, A. Niedzwiecki, M. Rath. *International Journal of Urology 2006; 13: 415-419*

Modulation of Human Renal Cell Carcinoma 786-0 MMP-2 and MMP-9 Activity by Inhibitors and Inducers in Vitro. M.W. Roomi, V. Ivanov, T. Kalinovsky, A. Niedzwiecki, M. Rath. *Medical Oncology 2006; 23(2): 245-250*

Anticancer Effect of Lysine, Proline, Arginine, Ascorbic Acid and Green Tea Extract on Human Renal Adenocarcinoma Line 786-0. M.W. Roomi, V. Ivanov, T. Kalinovsky, A. Niedzwiecki and M. Rath. *Oncology Reports 2006; 16(5):943-7*

SKIN CANCER

Inhibition of 7, 12-Dimethylbenzathracene-Induced Skin tumors by a Nutrient Mixture. M.W. Roomi, N.W. Roomi, T. Kalinovsky, V. Ivanov, M. Rath, A. Niedzwiecki. *Medical Oncology 2008; 25(3): 330-340*

Suppression of growth and hepatic metastasis of murine B16FO melanoma cells by a novel nutrient mixture. M.W. Roomi, T. Kalinovsky, N.W. Roomi, V. Ivanov, M. Rath, A. Niedzwiecki. *Oncology Reports 2008; 20:809-817*

In Vitro and In Vivo Antitumor Effect of Ascorbic Acid, Lysine, Proline, And Green Tea Extract On Human Melanoma Cell Line A2058. M.W. Roomi, V. Ivanov, T. Kalinovsky, A. Niedzwiecki, M. Rath. *In Vivo 2006;20(1): 25-32*

LUNG CANCER

Chemopreventive effect of a novel nutrient mixture on lung tumorigenesis induced by urethane in male A/J mice. M.W. Roomi, N.W. Roomi, V. Ivanov, T. Kalinovsky, A. Niedzwiecki, M. Rath. *Tumori 2009; 95: 508-513*

Modulation of MMP-2 and MMP-9 by cytokines, mitogens, and inhibitors in lung cancer and mesothelioma cell lines. M.W. Roomi, J.C. Monterrey, T. Kalinovsky, A. Niedzwiecki, M. Rath. *Oncology Reports 2009; 22: 1283-1291*

Inhibition of Malignant Mesothelioma Cell Matrix Metalloproteinase Production and Invasion by a Novel Nutrient mixture. M.W. Roomi, V. Ivanov, T. Kalinovsky, A. Niedzwiecki and M. Rath. *Experimental Lung Research 2006; 32:69-79*

In Vivo and in Vitro Anti-tumor Effect of a Unique Nutrient Mixture on Lung Cancer Cell Line A-549. M.W. Roomi, V. Ivanov, T. Kalinovsky, A. Niedzwiecki and M. Rath. *Experimental Lung Research 2006; 32:441-453*

Inhibition of Pulmonary Metastasis of Melanoma B16FO Cells in C57BL/6 Mice by a Nutrient Mixture Consisting of Ascorbic Acid, Lysine, Proline, Arginine, and Green Tea Extract. M.W. Roomi, V. Ivanov, T. Kalinovsky, A. Niedzwiecki, M. Rath *Experimental Lung Research 2006; 32(10):517-30*

BLOOD CANCER

Antineoplastic effect of nutrient mixture on Raji and Jurkat T cells: the two highly aggressive non-Hodgkin's lymphoma cell lines. M.W. Roomi, BA Bhanap, N.W. Roomi, A. Niedzwiecki and M. Rath. *Experimental Oncology 2009; 31(3): 149-155*

Epigallocatechin -3-Gallate induces apoptosis and cell cycle arrest in HTLV-1 positive and negative leukemia cells. S. Harakeh, K. Abu-El-Ardat, M. Diab-Assaf, A. Niedzwiecki, M. El-Sabban, M. Rath. *Medical Oncology 2008; 25: 30-39*

Ascorbic acid induces apoptosis in Adult T-cell Leukemia. S. Harakeh, M. Diab-Assaf, J. Khalife, K. Abu-El-Ardat, E. Baydoun, A. Niedzwiecki, M. El-Sabban, M. Rath. *Anticancer Research 2007; 27: 289-298*

Mechanistic aspects of apoptosis induction by L-Lysine in both HTLV-1 positive and negative cell lines. S. Harakeh, M. Diab-Assaf, K. Abu-El-Ardat, A. Niedzwiecki, M. Rath. *Chem. Biol. Interactions 2006; 164: 102-114*

Apoptosis Induction by Epican Forte in HTLV-1 Positive and Negative Malignant TCells. S. Harakeh, M. Diab-Assaf, A. Niedzwiecki, J. Khalife, K. Abu-El-Ardat, M. Rath. *Leukemia Research –2006; 30: 869-881*

OTHER TYPES OF CANCER

Comparative effects of EGCG, green tea and a nutrient mixture on the patterns of MMP-2 and MMP-9 expression in cancer cell lines. M.W. Roomi, J.C. Monterrey, T. Kalinovsky, A. Niedzwiecki, M. Rath. *Oncology Reports – 2010; 24:747-757*

Inhibition of invasion and MMPs by a nutrient mixture in human cancer cell lines: a correlation study. M.W. Roomi, J.C. Monterrey, T. Kalinovsky, A. Niedzwiecki, M. Rath. *Experimental Oncology- 2010; 32:243-248*

In vivo and in vitro effect of a nutrient mixture on human hepatocarcinoma cell line SK-Hep-1. M.W. Roomi, T. Kalinovsky, A. Niedzwiecki, M. Rath. *Experimental Oncology –2010;32:84-91*

Patterns of MMP-2 and MMP-9 expression in human cancer cell lines. M.W. Roomi, J.C. Monterrey, T. Kalinovsky, A. Niedzwiecki, M. Rath *Oncology Reports – 2009; 21:1323-1333*

Marked inhibition of growth and invasive parameters of head and neck squamous carcinoma FADU by a nutrient mixture. M.W. Roomi, N.W. Roomi, T. Kalinovsky, A. Niedzwiecki, M. Rath. *Integrative Cancer Therapies 2009; 8(2):168-176*

Inhibition of Glioma Cell Line A-172 MMP Activity and Cell Invasion in Vitro by a Nutrient Mixture. M.W. Roomi, V. Ivanov, T. Kalinovsky, A. Niedzwiecki and M. Rath. *Medical Oncology 2007; 24(2): 231-238*

Inhibitory of Cell Invasion and MMP Production by a Nutrient Mixture in Malignant Liposarcoma Cell Line SW-872. M.W. Roomi, V. Ivanov, T. Kalinovsky, A. Niedzwiecki, M. Rath. *Medical Oncology 2007; 24(4):394-401*

In Vitro Anticarcinogenic Effect of a Nutrient Mixture on Human Rhadomyosarcoma Cells. M.W. Roomi, V. Ivanov, T. Kalinovsky, A. Niedzwiecki, M. Rath *Gene Therapy and Molecular Biology 2007; 11(B):133-144*

In Vivo and in Vitro Anti-tumor Effect of a Nutrient Mixture Containing Ascorbic Acid, Lysine, Proline, and Green Tea Extract on Human Synovial Sarcoma Cancer Cells. M.W. Roomi, V. Ivanov, T. Kalinovsky, A. Niedzwiecki and M. Rath. *JAMA 2006; 9(2): 30-34*

A Specific Combination of Ascorbic Acid, Lysine, Proline and Epigallocatechin Gallate Inhibits Proliferation and Extracellular Matrix Invasion of Various Human Cancer Cell Lines. S.P. Netke, M.W. Roomi, V. Ivanov, A. Niedzwiecki, M. Rath. *Research Communications in Pharmacology and Toxicology, Emerging Drugs, 2003; Vol. II, IV37-IV50.*

METASTASIS

Micronutrient synergy – a new tool in effective control of metastasis and other key mechanisms of cancer. A. Niedzwiecki, M.W. Roomi, T. Kalinovsky, M. Rath. *Cancer Metastasis Review 2010; 29; 529-542*

Suppression of growth and hepatic metastasis of murine B16FO melanoma cells by a novel nutrient mixture. M.W. Roomi, T. Kalinovsky, N.W. Roomi, V. Ivanov, M. Rath, A. Niedzwiecki. *Oncology Reports 2008; 20:809-817*

A nutrient mixture suppresses hepatic metastasis in athymic nude mice injected with murine B16FO melanoma cells. M.W. Roomi, N.W. Roomi, T. Kalinovsky, J.C. Monterrery, M. Rath, and A. Niedzwiecki. *BioFactors 2008; 33; 85-97*

Inhibition of Pulmonary Metastasis of Melanoma B16FO Cells in C57BL/6 Mice by a Nutrient Mixture Consisting of Ascorbic Acid, Lysine, Proline, Arginine, and Green Tea Extract. M.W. Roomi, V. Ivanov, T. Kalinovsky, A. Niedzwiecki, M. Rath. *Experimental Lung Research 2006; 32(10):517-30*

ANGIOGENESIS
Distinct patterns of matrix metalloproteinase-2 and -9 expression in normal human cell lines. M.W. Roomi, J.C. Monterrery, T. Kalinovsky, M. Rath, and A. Niedzwiecki. *Oncology Reports – 2009; 21: 821-826*

Patterns of MMP-2 and MMP-9 expression in human cancer cell lines. M.W. Roomi, J.C. Monterrery, T. Kalinovsky, M. Rath, and A. Niedzwiecki. *Oncology Reports – 2009; 21:1323-1333*

Antiangiogenic properties of a nutrient mixture in a model of hemangioma. M.W. Roomi, T. Kalinovsky, M. Rath, and A. Niedzwiecki. *Experimental Oncology – Accepted 10/26/09*

A novel nutrient mixture containing ascorbic acid, lysine, proline and green tea extract inhibits critical parameters in angiogenesis . M.W. Roomi, V. Ivanov, T. Kalinovsky, A. Niedzwiecki, M. Rath in Anti-Angiogenic. Functional and Medicinal Foods, edited by Losso JN, Shahidi F, Bagchi D, *CRC Press, Taylor& Francis Group, Boca Raton, London, New York, 2007, pages 561-580.*

Inhibitory Effect of a Mixture Containing Ascorbic Acid, Lysine, Proline, and Green Tea Extract on Critical Parameters in Angiogenesis. M.W. Roomi, N.W. Roomi, V. Ivanov, T. Kalinovsky, A. Niedzwiecki, M. Rath. *Oncology Reports 2005, 14(4), 807-815.*

Antiangiogenic Effects of a Nutrient Mixture on Human Umbilical Vein Endothelial Cells. M.W. Roomi, N.W. Roomi, V. Ivanov, T. Kalinovsky, A. Niedzwiecki, M. Rath. *Oncology Reports 2005;14(6):1399-404*

Further references:

De Prithwish et al., Breast cancer incidence and hormone replacement therapy in Canada. *J. Natl. Cancer Inst. 2010; 102: 1-7*

Jemal A. et al., Global cancer statistics, *CA Cancer J Clin. 2011; 61: 69-90.*

Jemal A et al., Trends in the Leading Causes of Death in the United States, 1970-2002. *JAMA 2005, 294: 1255-1259*

Hirsh J, An Anniversary for Cancer Chemotherapy. *JAMA 2006; 296; 1518-1520.*

Phang J.M. et al., The metabolism of proline, a stress substance, modulates carcinogenic pathways. *Amino Acids, 2008; 35; 681-690*

Duffy M.J., The urokinase plasminogen activator system: role in malignancy. *Curr. Pharm. Des., 2004; 10; 39-49*

Henriet P et al., Contact with fibrillar collagen inhibits melanoma cell proliferation by up-regulating p27 KIP1. *Proc Natl Acad Sci USA, 2000; 97; 10026-10031.*

K. Almholt et al., Reduced metastasis of transgenic mammary cancer in urokinase deficient mice. *Int. J. Cancer 2005; 113: 525-532*

Ruhul Amin A.R.M. et al., Perspectives for Cancer Prevention with Natural Co pounds. *J. Clin. Oncol. 2009; 27: 2712-2725*

Oak Min-Ho et al., Antiangiogenic properties of natural polyphenols from red wine and green tea. *J. Nutr. Biochem. 2005; 16, 1-8*

Morgan G et al., The Contribution of Cytotoxic Chemotherapy to 5-year Survival in Adult Malignancies. *Clin. Oncol. 2004; 16: 549-560.*

Order information:

"Victory Over Cancer"

Part 1: Making the Unthinkable Possible
Part 2: Understanding History – Building the Future

Dr. Rath Health Foundation
1260 Memorex Drive, Suite 600
Santa Clara, CA 95030

Tel.: 866-367-8618
Fax: 408-748-1726

Email: info@drrath.com

Website: www.dr-rath-foundation.org

Matthias Rath, M.D. and
Aleksandra Niedzwiecki, Ph.D.

Victory
Over
Cancer!

Part 1:

Making the Unthinkable

Possible

Dr. Rath Health Foundation

Matthias Rath, M.D. and
Aleksandra Niedzwiecki, Ph.D.

Victory
Over
Cancer!

Part 2:

...ding History
...ng the Future

Dr. Rath Health Foundation

Important websites

While reading this book you probably encountered some topics that you want to know more about. Here is a collection of websites which we helped to build. We can guarantee that the contents of these sites are independent from the pharma business with disease:

- **www.drrathresearch.org**
  The official website of our research institute in California.

- **www.drrathresearch.org/research/publications/cancer.html**
  Direct link to the cancer studies of our research institue.

- **www.wha-www.org/en/library/index.html**
  Online library for health professionals who are engaged in natural therapies and patients.